The Clinical Neuroscience of Lateralization

The Clinical Neuroscience of Lateralization gives the first comprehensive transdiagnostic overview of the evidence for changes in hemispheric asymmetries in different psychiatric and neurodevelopmental disorders.

Taking a multidisciplinary perspective informed by both basic science and clinical studies, the authors integrate recent breakthroughs on hemispheric asymmetries in psychology, neuroscience, genetics, and comparative research. They give a general introduction to hemispheric asymmetries and the techniques used to assess them and review the evidence for changes in hemispheric asymmetries in different psychiatric and neurodevelopmental disorders. The book also discusses neurological disorders, like Parkinson's disease and multiple sclerosis, and highlights the importance of open science in clinical laterality research.

Offering a fresh perspective on a longstanding issue in clinical neuroscience, this book will be of great interest for academics, researchers, and students in the fields of clinical and developmental neuroscience, biopsychology, and neuropsychology.

Annakarina Mundorf is Postdoctoral Researcher at the Department of Medicine, Medical Psychology, MSH Medical School Hamburg, Germany.

Sebastian Ocklenburg is Professor of Biopsychology, Ruhr University Bochum, Germany.

The Clinical Neuroscience of Lateralization

**Annakarina Mundorf and
Sebastian Ocklenburg**

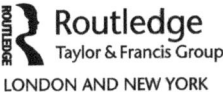

Routledge
Taylor & Francis Group

LONDON AND NEW YORK

First published 2021
by Routledge
2 Park Square, Milton Park, Abingdon, Oxon OX14 4RN

and by Routledge
605 Third Avenue, New York, NY 10158

Routledge is an imprint of the Taylor & Francis Group, an informa business

© 2021 **Annakarina Mundorf and Sebastian Ocklenburg**

British Library Cataloguing-in-Publication Data
A catalogue record for this book is available from the British Library

Library of Congress Cataloging-in-Publication Data
A catalog record has been requested for this book

ISBN: [9780367535797] (hbk)
ISBN: [9780367535810] (pbk)
ISBN: [9781003082507] (ebk)

Typeset in [Times New Roman]

For Helen Meyer and Jutta Peterburs.
Without you, our lives would be like a brain with only
one hemisphere—incomplete.

Contents

Foreword

14 January 2021
Asymmetry is the rule, rather than the exception in nature. From chiral molecules all the way to the morphology of living organisms and to the Baryon asymmetry in the universe, asymmetry is to be found in many levels and forms. *Homo sapiens* has certainly not escaped this fate and—as in all vertebrates—lateralization is a central principle of its nervous system. Laterality is thus an important field of enquiry for neuroscience researchers. Clinical neuroscience, the subfield of neuroscience that studies the fundamental mechanisms that underlie diseases and disorders of the nervous system, is in turn concerned with the investigation of laterality. An intriguing finding is that for each one of the neurodevelopmental and psychiatric disorders for which laterality data is available, asymmetries seem to be reduced on a population level compared to the general population. This realization is the driving force behind the writing of the book at hand.

The authors, Sebastian Ocklenburg, a leading international authority in the study of laterality, and Annakarina Mundorf, a promising young researcher in the field of clinical neuroscience, offer an informative, comprehensive, critical, and easy-to-follow overview of laterality research in the disorders of the nervous system. The first chapter introduces the reader to the concept of lateralization on the behavioural and the psychophysiological level as well as in terms of functional and structural hemispheric asymmetries. It further gives a short introduction to the relationship between laterality and neurodevelopmental and psychiatric disorders and briefly describes the main research methods employed in the field. Chapter 2 focuses on laterality in neurodevelopmental disorders. The third chapter discusses laterality findings in psychiatric disorders, while the fourth chapter summarizes the work that has been done in neurological disorders. And here comes the treat: the fifth chapter offers a theoretical integration of findings across disorders, discusses the biological pathways that overlap between the ontogenesis of hemispheric asymmetries and the pathogenesis of different disorders, and proposes a road map for future laterality research in clinical neuroscience: a transdiagnostic and symptom-based approach. Therefore, in this book, the authors do not simply organize and summarize research findings to date; they move on to develop a unified account, offering a deep and much-needed level of understanding of the literature.

The study of lateralization has seen an upsurge in publication in the last decades. McManus estimated that about 5,000 articles had been published on lateralization by 1985 (McManus 1986). Today, if one enters "laterality" as a key word in PubMed, nearly 392,000 hits will appear. This wealth of new information makes the work of even experienced researchers challenging. Keeping abreast of this exploding literature is not an easy feat, let alone finding the underlying knowledge that the results carry. Traditional literature reviews might be valuable but cannot make justice to such an abundance of data. Meta-analysis, by contrast, is a statistical method allowing for the statistical integration of the findings from a large collection of studies in a clear, objective manner. Meta-analysis further allows for the investigation of the presence of small study bias, allows for the assessment of any systematic variation among the results of different studies and, moreover, allows for the investigation of the sources of any such variance. I therefore consider it a central virtue of this book that the authors give weight to meta-analytic evidence, including both traditional meta-analyses as well as ALE meta-analyses. The authors further highlight the areas where meta-analytic integration is still needed, for example on dichotic listening data in the case of stuttering or on the relationship between depression and handedness. In addition to giving emphasis to evidence provided by meta-analyses, the authors underline the importance of conducting multi-lab studies and of analysing data coming from large databanks, such as the UK BioBank. Last but not least, the authors encourage researchers to apply open science principles in their work, such as pre-registering their studies and making data publicly available. All of these practices support the replicability of research: an essential quality of solid scientific research.

This book was a pleasure to read. It is written in a manner that is friendly both for the expert in laterality as well as the non-expert reader. I learned a lot and consider myself richer for that. I was expecting nothing less from Sebastian and Annakarina.

Marietta Papadatou-Pastou

Assistant Professor

National and Kapodistrian University of Athens

Biomedical Research Foundation Academy of Athens

McManus, I.C., 1986. Book review: left side, right side: a review of laterality research (Beaton, A.). *British Journal of Psychology*, 77, 419–421.

Preface

The human brain is one of the most complex entities in the known universe. We are the only species that writes love letters, tax declarations, or Nobel Prize-winning novels. These amazing abilities do come at a price, though. High complexity often begets a certain fragility. While the human brain is capable of creating amazing works of art, it is also vulnerable to mental illness to an extent that is unmatched in any other species.

Whether someone develops mental health issues or not has been investigated from several different research perspectives. With this book, we hope to give a comprehensive review of ongoing trends and perspectives on the link between neurodevelopmental, psychiatric, and neurological disorders as well as one particularly important aspect of brain organization: hemispheric asymmetries. Thus, allowing researchers of different backgrounds to investigate the clinical neuroscience of laterality as an integrated view on the topic is highly needed to further advance the field.

As often in life, the sum is more than its parts when it comes to writing a book. The two hemispheres of our brains have different specializations. Connected by the corpus callosum, they work together millions of times every day to ensure coordinated behaviour in interaction with the environment. This book came into existence in a similar fashion. Two scientists coming from quite different backgrounds working together, united by a common vision and the love for science. We hope that by combining Annakarina's strong neurobiological comparative psychiatry perspective with Sebastian's roots in laterality research in humans, we were able offer a new perspective on clinical laterality research: one that has been updated from previous efforts to reflect the rapid developments in this exiting field.

Bochum, Germany, January 2021
Annakarina Mundorf and Sebastian Ocklenburg

Acknowledgements

This book would not have been possible without the help of several individuals. In particular, we would like to give our heartfelt thanks to Stephanie Lor, Judith Schmitz, and Jutta Peterburs for critical comments on our initial drafts. Moreover, we would like to thank Marietta Papadatou-Pastou (a.k.a. the queen of laterality meta-analyses) for writing the foreword for our book. Additionally, we would like to thank the editorial team at Routledge for their dedication and support—without their help, this book would not have been possible.

1 Lateralization in neurodevelopmental, psychiatric, and neurological disorders

Introduction

> All mental processes are brain processes, and therefore all disorders of mental functioning are biological diseases.
>
> Eric Kandel (cited in Weir 2012)

This statement by Nobel Prize laureate Eric Kandel exemplifies the key assumption of modern clinical neuroscience: the roots of mental illness lie in the disruption of biological processes in the brain. This implies that, in order to understand mental illness, it is crucial to understand how and why patients suffering from mental health problems show differences in brain organization compared to healthy individuals.

One of the most important organizational features of the human brain (or any vertebrate brain for that matter) is its division into two halves, or hemispheres (Ocklenburg and Güntürkün 2018). While looking mostly symmetrical on the macrostructural level, the two hemispheres show countless left-right differences, so-called hemispheric asymmetries (see next section). Among the most intriguing empirical findings related to these hemispheric asymmetries is the fact that they show alterations in almost all of the investigated psychiatric and neurodevelopmental disorders (Ocklenburg *et al.* 2015). These include—to name the most common examples—dyslexia (Paracchini *et al.* 2016), schizophrenia (Gruzelier 1984), affective disorders (Hecht 2010), autism spectrum disorders (Lindell and Hudry 2013), post-traumatic stress disorder (Meyer *et al.* 2015), attention deficit hyperactivity disorder (Lin and Tsuang 2018), and alcohol use disorder (Zhu *et al.* 2018).

Despite the wealth of the published literature (there are several hundred scientific papers on hemispheric asymmetries in schizophrenia alone), the relationship between hemispheric asymmetries and psychiatric and neurodevelopmental disorders is still far from being well understood. In particular, most empirical papers focus on hemispheric asymmetries in one specific disorder, but there rarely is an overarching integration of findings across different disorders. Therefore, the present book aims to not only review empirical findings on functional and structural hemispheric asymmetries in these and other disorders but also to integrate these findings across disorders. Moreover, we aim to synthesize the findings of the biological pathways that overlap between the ontogenesis of hemispheric asymmetries and the pathogenesis of different disorders.

The book will start with a short definition of the relevant terminology in Chapter 1, followed by chapters reviewing the literature on hemispheric asymmetries in neurodevelopmental, psychiatric, and neurological disorders. The book will conclude with a chapter integrating results found in the different disorders and discussing the causality of the relation between hemispheric asymmetries and presented disorders.

What are hemispheric asymmetries?

The term hemispheric asymmetry generally describes functional or structural left-right differences in the brain. Typically, the hemisphere that is faster or more accurate for a specific cognitive function is called the dominant hemisphere. In contrast, the other hemisphere is called the non-dominant hemisphere. Hemispheric asymmetries are typically relative. Even if one hemisphere is dominant for a specific cognitive task, the other side of the brain is typically also active to some extent.

Hemispheric asymmetries have been described in several functional domains. In neuroscience, the most widely investigated forms of functional hemispheric asymmetries include handedness (Michel *et al.* 2018; Schmitz *et al.* 2017; Uomini and Ruck 2018), language lateralization (Corballis 2015; Hodgson and Hudson 2018; Ocklenburg *et al.* 2014), and emotional lateralization (Kotz *et al.* 2006; Lindell 2018; Wildgruber *et al.* 2006). In addition to these cognitive domains, functional hemispheric asymmetries have been described in many other brain functions. These include for example pro- and antisocial tendencies (Hecht 2014), memory (Moorman and Nicol 2015), visuospatial abilities (Dieterich and Brandt 2018), face perception (Frässle *et al.* 2016), arithmetic processing (Pinel and Dehaene 2010), and music processing (Limb 2006). On the structural level, hemispheric asymmetries have been described on the macrostructural, microstructural, and gene expression level (Amunts 2010). The most prominent examples of structural hemispheric asymmetries in the human brain include leftward asymmetry of the planum temporale (Shapleske *et al.* 1999) and leftward asymmetry of the arcuate fasciculus (Ocklenburg *et al.* 2016).

Importantly, not all individuals show the same hemispheric asymmetries, but there are varying levels of interindividual differences for different forms of hemispheric asymmetries. For example, for language lateralization, most individuals show stronger activations in the left hemisphere when processing language (Hugdahl and Westerhausen 2016), even though there are also some specific contributions of the right hemisphere, for example, to processing the emotional prosody of spoken language (Mitchell and Crow 2005). However, not all individuals show leftward language lateralization. It has been shown that in about 4% of strong right-handers, 15% of ambidextrous individuals, and 27% of strong left-handers, the right hemisphere is dominant for language processing (Knecht *et al.* 2000). Based on the relative prevalence of right- and left-hemispheric dominance across the population, it can be determined whether an individual shows typical (e.g. leftward language lateralization) or atypical (e.g. rightward language lateralization) lateralization for a specific cognitive function.

Atypical hemispheric asymmetries in neurodevelopmental, psychiatric, and neurological disorders

The core finding that inspired the conception of this book is the fact that, for all neurodevelopmental, psychiatric, and neurological disorders in which hemispheric asymmetries have been investigated to date, there is evidence for a higher prevalence of atypical hemispheric asymmetries than in the general population (see following chapters for details). In contrast, not a single disorder has been associated with a consistently higher prevalence of typical hemispheric asymmetries. Over the years, many different and somewhat diverging claims have been made about this intriguing observation. These can be differentiated into theories stating that atypical hemispheric asymmetries are the cause of mental illness, its consequence, or a correlate (Bishop 2013):

- Cause: For example, in the field of schizophrenia research, Crow and co-workers claimed that there is a causal relationship between atypical hemispheric asymmetries and the development of psychosis (Angrilli *et al.* 2009; Crow 1997, 2000). Specifically, they argued that people lacking left-hemispheric language dominance have an increased risk to develop schizophrenia, in particular positive symptoms such as auditory hallucinations and delusions (Angrilli *et al.* 2009).
- Correlate: An example of the theory that atypical hemispheric asymmetries might represent a correlate of mental illness also comes from

schizophrenia research. Oertel-Knochel and co-workers suggested that atypical structural and functional asymmetries represent a biomarker for schizophrenia, rather than a causal factor leading to psychosis (Oertel-Knochel *et al.* 2012).

• Consequence: Last but not least, an example of the idea that altered hemispheric asymmetries are a consequence, rather than cause or correlate, comes from dyslexia research. Here, Bishop suggested that atypical non-left language lateralization is a consequence rather than the cause of dyslexia (Bishop 2013) (see Chapter 5 for a more in-depth discussion of these ideas).

The investigation of the relations between atypical lateralization and neurodevelopmental, psychiatric, and neurological disorders has a long history in laterality research. In his book, *On the Other Hand: Left Hand, Right Brain, Mental Disorder, and History*, Harold I. Kushner gave a comprehensive overview of the main historical roots for the relationship between hemispheric asymmetries and pathology (Kushner 2017). We will highlight the most important ideas in the respective sections about specific disorders, but readers interested in a complete in-depth analysis of historical developments are kindly referred to this excellent work.

At the beginning of the 2020s, clinical laterality research is at a crossroad. Psychology and neuroscience are facing a so-called "replication crisis", as many results from smaller studies with low statistical power do not replicate when the experiment is again conducted in another lab (Anderson and Maxwell 2017). In the context of this replication crisis, not only studies with small samples face increasing scrutiny. Additionally, potentially overblown interpretations of the results of these studies are seen more critically than used to be the case. Laterality research is no exception here. For example, one of the core problems with all claims that atypical lateralization causes schizophrenia or other forms of mental illness is the fact that there is a large number of healthy individuals with atypical lateralization. For example, most left-handers or most people with rightward language lateralization do not develop any disorder (Cai *et al.* 2013; van der Haegen *et al.* 2013). Any claims that altered hemispheric asymmetries are the cause of any disorders need to have a convincing explanation for this finding, and typically, this is not the case. Thus, such claims need to be interpreted cautiously. Throughout the book, we will therefore critically evaluate any claims about the relationship of hemispheric asymmetries and specific disorders and will try (as Mike Corballis has put it) to differentiate "facts from fantasies" (Corballis 2014). Another important recent development in laterality research is the increasing amount of large-scale multi-centre studies in genetics and neuroimaging that include data on both hemispheric asymmetries and clinical parameters. Among these are, for example, the ENIGMA consortium (De Kong *et al.* 2018, 2019) and the UK Biobank (Carrion-Castillo *et al.* 2020; de Kovel and Francks 2019). Since these datasets include larger cohorts than almost all previous clinical laterality studies, we will take care to highlight their implications in detail in the respective chapters.

Techniques to assess hemispheric asymmetries

A wide variety of methods have been used to assess hemispheric asymmetries in both humans and non-human species. A recent book by Rogers and Vallortigara, entitled *Lateralized Brain Functions: Methods in Human and Non-Human Species*, described the most widely used techniques in laterality research on more than 700 pages (Rogers and Vallortigara 2017). This book represents an excellent resource for any researcher in need of detailed information about how to investigate hemispheric asymmetries. For the sake of brevity, we will only give a short overview of the main techniques that have been used in clinical laterality research in the present volume.

Questionnaires

Behavioural left-right preferences like handedness, footedness, or side preferences in ear and eye used are often assessed with questionnaires. Well-known examples include the Edinburgh Handedness Inventory (Oldfield 1971) and newer handedness questionnaires developed based on it (Veale 2014), or the Waterloo Footedness Questionnaire (Elias and Bryden 1998; Elias *et al.* 1998). Typically, these questionnaires include a number of items asking about the participant's limb or sensory organ that is preferentially used for several tasks such as writing, drawing, or opening a lid for handedness. Based on an individual's distribution of right and left answers, the experimenter can determine a laterality quotient (LQ) that indicates both direction and strength of the participant's preference. Typically, the LQ ranges between -100 (consistent left-sided preference) and +100 (consistent right-sided preference).

Neuropsychological tests

In addition to questionnaires, several neuropsychological tests have been used to assess hemispheric asymmetries on the behavioural level. For example, a commonly used behavioural task to measure hand skill is the so-called pegboard or peg-moving task (Annett 1976; Eling 1983). In this simple task, participants sit in front of a board that has two rows of holes in it. They are instructed to move several wooden pegs (usually ten) from one row to the other as fast as possible. The time needed to move all pegs from one row to the other is used as the dependent variable, and by comparing the performance of the left and the right hand over several trials, the more skilled hand can be identified.

Another widely used neuropsychological test in laterality research is the line bisection task (Jewell and McCourt 2000). In this task, a sheet of paper with lines of different lengths at different positions is presented to the participant. The participant is asked to bisect the line exactly in the middle. While patients with neglect (i.e. attentional deficits due to brain lesions) often show a rightward bisection error, healthy participants often show a leftward bisection error (Friedrich *et al.* 2018). This leftward bisection error is thought to reflect right-hemispheric dominance for visuospatial processing.

Psychophysiological paradigms

Psychophysiological paradigms in which reaction times and accuracy rates to experimentally presented stimuli (e.g. visual shapes on a computer monitor or spoken syllables on headphones) are assessed have a long history in laterality research. One of the most widely used acoustic paradigms in clinical laterality research is the so-called dichotic listening task (Hugdahl 2000; Tervaniemi and Hugdahl 2003; Westerhausen and Kompus 2018). In this task, participants wear headphones and listen to two different acoustic stimuli (e.g. words or syllables) that are presented simultaneously to the left and the right ear. They are then asked to indicate which stimulus they heard best. Typically, most participants show a right ear advantage, meaning that they report more of the stimuli presented to the right ear than of the stimuli presented to the left ear. This is thought to reflect left-hemispheric dominance for the processing of acoustic speech stimuli (Westerhausen 2019). One commonly used variant of the classic dichotic listening task is the forced attention dichotic listening task (Hugdahl *et al.* 2009). In this variant of the task, participants are tested in two additional conditions. In the "forced right" condition, they are instructed to only attend to stimuli presented to the right ear, and in the "forced left" condition, they are asked to only attend to stimuli presented to the left ear. These additional conditions allow for the assessment of the effects of cognitive control on hemispheric asymmetries (Westerhausen *et al.* 2015).

Another widely used family of psychophysical paradigms in research on hemispheric asymmetries are experiments based on the so-called visual half-field technique (Bourne 2006). Here, participants are asked to fixate a fixation cross in the middle of a screen while seated at a specific viewing distance from this screen. Then, visual stimuli are shown tachistoscopically, that is, so fast that no information transfer to the other hemisphere over the corpus callosum takes place. The idea is that when participants are now asked to react to the presented stimulus, it is only or mostly processed by the hemisphere contralateral to the visual field in which the stimulus was presented. As fixation of the fixation cross is essential for this principle to work, it is often advised to control eye movement using an eye tracker. Typically, participants react faster and more accurately to stimuli presented in the visual hemifield contralateral to the dominant hemisphere for a specific stimulus type. The visual half-field technique has successfully been used to assess hemispheric asymmetries in several different cognitive domains, including language processing (De Clercq and Brysbaert 2020), visuospatial processing (Hausmann and Güntürkün 1999), and face processing (Gerrits *et al.* 2019).

Functional hemispheric asymmetries in electrophysiological activity

Electroencephalography (EEG) is used to measure electric activity on the scalp using a set of electrodes and amplifying it (Luck 2014). EEG data can be analysed in several different ways, but there are two main applications in clinical neuroscience.

First, asymmetries in oscillations in different frequency bands that can be extracted from the EEG raw signal have been of interest (Herrmann *et al.* 2016). Here, particularly frontal asymmetries in the alpha band (8–12 Hz) have been the focus of clinical laterality research (Allen *et al.* 2018; Reznik and Allen 2018). Activity in the alpha band has been thought of as a marker for the absence of cognitive activity so that a rightward asymmetry in alpha band activity would indicate greater cognitive activity in the left hemisphere. Importantly, some clinical groups, such as patients with depression, show a leftward shift of EEG alpha band power compared to healthy controls indicating greater right-frontal than left-frontal cortical activity (see the section on hemispheric asymmetries in affective disorders for more information).

Second, asymmetries in so-called event-related potentials (ERPs) have been investigated in clinical laterality research. ERPs are the mean electrophysiological responses to a specific event such as stimulus or response onset. For example, both asymmetries in early components of the stimulus-locked ERP, such as the P1, N1, and P2 as well as late ERP components like the P3, have been investigated in patients suffering from affective disorders (Baskaran *et al.* 2012; Monnart *et al.* 2016; Trinkl *et al.* 2015).

Functional hemispheric asymmetries in brain activation

The most commonly used technique to assess functional hemispheric asymmetries in brain activation is functional magnetic resonance imaging (fMRI) (Huettel *et al.* 2014). In general, fMRI estimates activity in specific brain areas by measuring the flow of oxygenated blood in the brain. By comparing brain activation in homologous brain areas in the left and the right hemisphere during a specific cognitive task, the extent of hemispheric asymmetry for a specific cognitive domain can be assessed. For example, fMRI has been used to assess functional hemispheric asymmetries for language processing (Hugdahl and Westerhausen 2016), face perception (Bukowski *et al.* 2013), visuospatial abilities (Zago *et al.* 2017), and many others. Moreover, resting state fMRI has been used in various clinical groups to assess hemispheric asymmetries in resting state networks such as the default mode network (Li *et al.* 2018).

In addition to fMRI, several other techniques have been used to assess hemispheric asymmetries in brain activation. These include for example functional transcranial Doppler sonography (Deppe *et al.* 2004; Lohmann *et al.* 2005; Knecht *et al.* 2000), positron emission tomography (PET) (Savic and Lindström 2008; Zahn *et al.* 2004; Zhou *et al.* 2009), and functional near-infrared spectroscopy (fNIRS) (Cai *et al.* 2019).

Structural hemispheric asymmetries in grey matter

Magnetic resonance imaging (MRI) is the most widely used technique to assess structural hemispheric asymmetries in grey matter (e.g. in volume, shape, surface area, or depth of different grey matter areas) (Elnakib *et al.* 2014). By comparing these parameters between homologous brain areas in the left and right hemisphere, the extent of structural hemispheric asymmetry can be determined. One commonly used method to assess group differences in the local concentration of grey matter between patients and healthy controls is voxel-based morphometry (VBM) (Ashburner and Friston 2000). Here, a specific workflow to assess hemispheric asymmetries has recently been proposed (Kurth *et al.* 2015). MRI has been used to assess structural asymmetries in almost all clinical groups discussed in this book, and the results will be given in detail in the respective chapters.

Structural hemispheric asymmetries in white matter

Diffusion tensor imaging (DTI) is the most widely used technique to assess structural hemispheric asymmetries in white matter (Tournier and Mori 2014). In clinical laterality research, two main ways to analyse hemispheric asymmetries in white matter structure are commonly used. First, probabilistic or deterministic tractography (Mukherjee *et al.* 2008a, 2008b) is used to assess structural asymmetries of specific white matter tracts like the arcuate fasciculus, uncinate fasciculus, or superior longitudinal fasciculus. For example, leftward asymmetry in fractional anisotropy in the arcuate fasciculus, a major white matter tract in the language system, has been identified using tractography (Nucifora *et al.* 2005). Another commonly used method to analyse asymmetries in the white matter based on DTI data is tract-based spatial statistics (TBSS) (Smith *et al.* 2006). Here, asymmetries are not analysed based on specific white matter tracts that are neuroanatomically defined, but for each voxel separately, allowing for a finer-grained analysis of asymmetries in subparts of larger tracts (Takao *et al.* 2011; Ocklenburg *et al.* 2013).

Structural hemispheric asymmetries in neurite structure

Another form of diffusion imaging that has been used in research on structural hemispheric asymmetries is neurite orientation dispersion and density imaging (NODDI) (Ocklenburg *et al.* 2018; Schmitz *et al.* 2019a, 2019b). NODDI allows for the assessment of asymmetries in microstructural complexity of axons and dendrites in both grey and white matter (Zhang *et al.* 2012). Recent research suggests that these microstructural asymmetries might have stronger associations with electrophysiological asymmetries than macrostructural measures of hemispheric asymmetries obtained from standard MRI. While NODDI has not yet been used to investigate hemispheric asymmetries in clinical samples, it is a promising technique that will likely be used in the field in the coming decade.

Psychiatric, neurodevelopmental, and neurological disorders

As mentioned previously, one of the most intriguing findings in laterality research is the fact that in many psychiatric and neurodevelopmental disorders, patients show a higher prevalence of atypical hemispheric asymmetries than the general population. Here, we would like to give a short overview of the disorders covered in this book.

In general, there are two different systems for diagnosing psychiatric disorders: The Diagnostic and Statistical Manual of Mental Disorders, 5th Edition (DSM-5), and the International Classification of Diseases, Tenth Revision (ICD-10). The ICD-10 is the official standard diagnostic tool for mental health provided by the World Health Organization (WHO 2016).

Regarding the diagnosis of schizophrenia, for example, the two systems overlap to a large extent. The DSM-5 gives more weight to social dysfunction than the ICD-10, whereas the ICD-10 puts more emphasis on first-rank (psychiatric) symptoms occurring in schizophrenia (American Psychiatric Association 2013; Jakobsen *et al.* 2005). In this book, we will use both systems, but the focus will lie on the DSM-5. Generally, a mental disorder is defined by clinically noticeable disturbances in personal cognition, emotion regulation, or when behaviour mediated by mental functioning is to some extent dysfunctional, leading to deficits in everyday life (American Psychiatric Association 2013). For example, mental disorders are marked by an exaggeration of normal behaviour (e.g. negative affect is exaggerated in depression, feelings of euphoria occur excessively in manic episodes of bipolar disorder, normal fear is overwhelming in anxiety disorders). In contrast, neurological diseases produce unusual behaviour such as uncontrolled body movement in Parkinson's disease. Moreover, neurological, and mental disorders both show reduced neural function, such as reduced cognition observed in schizophrenia, reduced social skills in autism spectrum disorder, and reduced memory in Alzheimer's disease. However, these disorders are not only associated with a reduction in skills but sometimes also with, for example, extraordinary creativity as can be observed in some people diagnosed with schizophrenia, bipolar disorder, and autism spectrum disorder.

In the following chapters, we will discuss atypical lateralization and the neurodevelopmental disorders dyslexia, autism spectrum disorders, stuttering, and attention deficit hyperactivity disorder. Neurodevelopmental disorders are characterized by an early manifestation of developmental deficits in the emotional, social, personal, or academic life of the affected child. Moreover, they often have a highly hereditary (genetic) aetiology.

In terms of psychiatric disorders, we will discuss atypical lateralization and schizophrenia, affective disorders, substance-related and addictive disorders, and posttraumatic stress disorder. Symptomatically, these disorders have fewer common characteristics, but they are usually all manifesting during late adolescence or early adulthood and share a rather highly environmental aetiology with lesser-known genetic risk variants.

As a third category of disorders, we will sum up findings of atypical lateralization and the neurological disorders Parkinson's disease, Alzheimer's disease, and multiple sclerosis. In general, neuronal degeneration also implies the loss of function. Thus, these disorders are associated with a progressive reduction of neurons, synaptic plasticity, and other neuronal processes in common, leading to physical problems such as loss of motor control and cognitive problems like memory loss and reduced executive functions. Except for multiple sclerosis, most of the neurological disorders manifest later in adult life and often have a highly genetic aetiology.

John Hughlings Jackson (1835–1911) was the first to state that the left hemisphere inhibits the right so that damage to the left hemisphere might enhance creativity (Kandel 2018). He also assumed that when the left hemisphere is compromised, the right hemisphere becomes dominant, resulting in difficulties in speech, as in dyslexia. Thus, John Hughlings Jackson was one of the first scientists to suggest an association between lateralization and psychiatric disorders. Following these early ideas, a vast number of studies on lateralization have been conducted in different patient groups. Today, the clinical neuroscience of lateralization is a thriving research field and with this book, we hope to give an up-to-date overview of recent trends and developments in the field.

References

Allen, J.J.B., *et al.*, 2018. Frontal EEG alpha asymmetry and emotion: from neural underpinnings and methodological considerations to psychopathology and social cognition. *Psychophysiology*, 55 (1).

American Psychiatric Association, 2013. *Diagnostic and statistical manual of mental disorders. DSM-5.* 5th ed. Washington, DC: American Psychiatric Publishing.

Amunts, C., 2010. Structural indices of asymmetry. *In:* K. Hugdahl and R. Westerhausen, eds. *The two halves of the brain.* Cambridge, MA: The MIT Press, 145–176.

Anderson, S.F., and Maxwell, S.E., 2017. Addressing the "replication crisis": using original studies to design replication studies with appropriate statistical power. *Multivariate Behavioral Research*, 52 (3), 305–324.

Angrilli, A., *et al.*, 2009. Schizophrenia as failure of left hemispheric dominance for the phonological component of language. *PLoS One*, 4 (2), e4507.

Annett, M., 1976. A coordination of hand preference and skill replicated. *British Journal of Psychology (London, England: 1953)*, 67 (4), 587–592.

Ashburner, J., and Friston, K.J., 2000. Voxel-based morphometry—the methods. *NeuroImage*, 11 (6 Pt 1), 805–821.

Baskaran, A., Milev, R., and McIntyre, R.S., 2012. The neurobiology of the EEG biomarker as a predictor of treatment response in depression. *Neuropharmacology*, 63 (4), 507–513.

Bishop, D.V.M., 2013. Cerebral asymmetry and language development: cause, correlate, or consequence? *Science (New York, N.Y.)*, 340 (6138), 1230531.

Bourne, V.J., 2006. The divided visual field paradigm: methodological considerations. *Laterality*, 11 (4), 373–393.

Bukowski, H., *et al.*, 2013. Cerebral lateralization of face-sensitive areas in left-handers: only the FFA does not get it right. *Cortex; A Journal Devoted to the Study of the Nervous System and Behavior*, 49 (9), 2583–2589.

Cai, L., *et al.*, 2019. Functional near-infrared spectroscopy evidence for the development of topological asymmetry between hemispheric brain networks from childhood to adulthood. *Neurophotonics*, 6 (2), 25005.

Cai, Q., van der Haegen, L., and Brysbaert, M., 2013. Complementary hemispheric specialization for language production and visuospatial attention. *Proceedings of the National Academy of Sciences of the United States of America*, 110 (4), E322–E330.

Carrion-Castillo, A., *et al.*, 2020. Genetic effects on planum temporale asymmetry and their limited relevance to neurodevelopmental disorders, intelligence or educational attainment. *Cortex; a Journal Devoted to the Study of the Nervous System and Behavior*, 124, 137–153.

Corballis, M.C., 2014. Left brain, right brain: facts and fantasies. *PLoS Biology*, 12 (1), e1001767.

Corballis, M.C., 2015. What's left in language? Beyond the classical model. *Annals of the New York Academy of Sciences*, 1359, 14–29.

Crow, T.J., 1997. Schizophrenia as failure of hemispheric dominance for language. *Trends in Neurosciences*, 20 (8), 339–343.

Crow, T.J., 2000. Schizophrenia as the price that homo sapiens pays for language: a resolution of the central paradox in the origin of the species. *Brain Research. Brain Research Reviews*, 31 (2–3), 118–129.

De Clercq, P., and Brysbaert, M., 2020. The influence of word valence on the right visual field advantage in the VHF paradigm: time to adjust the expectations. *Laterality*, 25, 537–559.

De Kovel, C.G.F., *et al.*, 2019. No alterations of brain structural asymmetry in major depressive disorder: an ENIGMA consortium analysis. *The American Journal of Psychiatry*, 176 (12), 1039–1049.

De Kovel, C.G.F., and Francks, C., 2019. The molecular genetics of hand preference revisited. *Scientific Reports*, 9 (1), 5986.

Deppe, M., Ringelstein, E.B., and Knecht, S., 2004. The investigation of functional brain lateralization by transcranial Doppler sonography. *NeuroImage*, 21 (3), 1124–1146.

Dieterich, M., and Brandt, T., 2018. Global orientation in space and the lateralization of brain functions. *Current Opinion in Neurology*, 31 (1), 96–104.

Elias, L.J., and Bryden, M.P., 1998. Footedness is a better predictor of language lateralisation than handedness. *Laterality*, 3 (1), 41–51.

Elias, L.J., Bryden, M.P., and Bulman-Fleming, M.B., 1998. Footedness is a better predictor than is handedness of emotional lateralization. *Neuropsychologia*, 36 (1), 37–43.

Eling, P., 1983. Comparing different measures of laterality: do they relate to a single mechanism? *Journal of Clinical Neuropsychology*, 5 (2), 135–147.

Elnakib, A., *et al.*, 2014. Magnetic resonance imaging findings for dyslexia: a review. *Journal of Biomedical Nanotechnology*, 10 (10), 2778–2805.

Frässle, S., *et al.*, 2016. Mechanisms of hemispheric lateralization: asymmetric interhemispheric recruitment in the face perception network. *NeuroImage*, 124 (Pt A), 977–988.

Friedrich, T.E., Hunter, P.V., and Elias, L.J., 2018. The trajectory of pseudoneglect in adults: a systematic review. *Neuropsychology Review*, 28 (4), 436–452.

Gerrits, R., *et al.*, 2019. Laterality for recognizing written words and faces in the fusiform gyrus covaries with language dominance. *Cortex; a Journal Devoted to the Study of the Nervous System and Behavior*, 117, 196–204.

Gruzelier, J.H., 1984. Hemispheric imbalances in schizophrenia. *International Journal of Psychophysiology: Official Journal of the International Organization of Psychophysiology*, 1 (3), 227–240.

Hausmann, M., and Güntürkün, O., 1999. Sex differences in functional cerebral asymmetries in a repeated measures design. *Brain and Cognition*, 41 (3), 263–275.

Hecht, D., 2010. Depression and the hyperactive right-hemisphere. *Neuroscience Research*, 68 (2), 77–87.

Hecht, D., 2014. Cerebral lateralization of pro- and anti-social tendencies. *Experimental Neurobiology*, 23 (1), 1–27.

Herrmann, C.S., *et al.*, 2016. EEG oscillations: from correlation to causality. *International Journal of Psychophysiology: Official Journal of the International Organization of Psychophysiology*, 103, 12–21.

Hodgson, J.C., and Hudson, J.M., 2018. Speech lateralization and motor control. *Progress in Brain Research*, 238, 145–178.

Huettel, S.A., Song, A.W., and McCarthy, G., 2014. *Functional magnetic resonance imaging*. Sunderland, MA: Sinauer Associates. Inc. Publishers.

Hugdahl, K., 2000. Lateralization of cognitive processes in the brain. *Acta Psychologica*, 105 (2–3), 211–235.

Hugdahl, K., *et al.*, 2009. Attention and cognitive control: unfolding the dichotic listening story. *Scandinavian Journal of Psychology*, 50 (1), 11–22.

Hugdahl, K., and Westerhausen, R., 2016. Speech processing asymmetry revealed by dichotic listening and functional brain imaging. *Neuropsychologia*, 93 (Pt B), 466–481.

Jakobsen, K.D., *et al.*, 2005. Reliability of clinical ICD-10 schizophrenia diagnoses. *Nordic Journal of Psychiatry*, 59 (3), 209–212.

Jewell, G., and McCourt, M.E., 2000. Pseudoneglect: a review and meta-analysis of performance factors in line bisection tasks. *Neuropsychologia*, 38 (1), 93–110.

Kandel, E.R., 2018. *The disordered mind. What unusual brains tell us about ourselves*. New York: Farrar, Strauss and Giroux.

Knecht, S., *et al.*, 2000. Handedness and hemispheric language dominance in healthy humans. *Brain: A Journal of Neurology*, 123 (Pt 12), 2512–2518.

Kong, X.-Z., *et al.*, 2018. Mapping cortical brain asymmetry in 17,141 healthy individuals worldwide via the ENIGMA consortium. *Proceedings of the National Academy of Sciences of the United States of America*, 115 (22), E5154–E5163.

Kotz, S.A., Meyer, M., and Paulmann, S., 2006. Lateralization of emotional prosody in the brain: an overview and synopsis on the impact of study design. *Progress in Brain Research*, 156, 285–294.

Kurth, F., Gaser, C., and Luders, E., 2015. A 12-step user guide for analyzing voxelwise gray matter asymmetries in statistical parametric mapping (SPM). *Nature Protocols*, 10 (2), 293–304.

Kushner, H.I., 2017. *On the other hand. Left hand, right brain, mental disorder, and history*. Baltimore, MD: Johns Hopkins University Press.

Li, G., *et al.*, 2018. Resting-state brain activity in Chinese boys with low functioning autism spectrum disorder. *Annals of General Psychiatry*, 17, 47.

Limb, C.J., 2006. Structural and functional neural correlates of music perception. *The Anatomical Record. Part A, Discoveries in Molecular, Cellular, and Evolutionary Biology*, 288 (4), 435–446.

Lin, H.-L., and Tsuang, H.-C., 2018. Handedness and attention deficit/hyperactivity disorder symptoms in college students. *The Psychiatric Quarterly*, 89 (1), 103–110.

Lindell, A.K., 2018. Lateralization of the expression of facial emotion in humans. *Progress in Brain Research*, 238, 249–270.

Lindell, A.K., and Hudry, K., 2013. Atypicalities in cortical structure, handedness, and functional lateralization for language in autism spectrum disorders. *Neuropsychology Review*, 23 (3), 257–270.

Lohmann, H., *et al.*, 2005. Language lateralization in young children assessed by functional transcranial Doppler sonography. *NeuroImage*, 24 (3), 780–790.

Luck, S.J., 2014. *An introduction to the event-related potential technique.* Cambridge, MA and London, England: The MIT Press.

Meyer, T., *et al.*, 2015. The role of frontal EEG asymmetry in post-traumatic stress disorder. *Biological Psychology*, 108, 62–77.

Michel, G.F., *et al.*, 2018. Evolution and development of handedness: an Evo-Devo approach. *Progress in Brain Research*, 238, 347–374.

Mitchell, R.L.C., and Crow, T.J., 2005. Right hemisphere language functions and schizophrenia: the forgotten hemisphere? *Brain: A Journal of Neurology*, 128 (Pt 5), 963–978.

Monnart, A., *et al.*, 2016. Just swap out of negative vibes? Rumination and inhibition deficits in major depressive disorder: data from event-related potentials studies. *Frontiers in Psychology*, 7, 1019.

Moorman, S., and Nicol, A.U., 2015. Memory-related brain lateralisation in birds and humans. *Neuroscience and Biobehavioral Reviews*, 50, 86–102.

Mukherjee, P., *et al.*, 2008a. Diffusion tensor MR imaging and fiber tractography: technical considerations. *AJNR. American Journal of Neuroradiology*, 29 (5), 843–852.

Mukherjee, P., *et al.*, 2008b. Diffusion tensor MR imaging and fiber tractography: theoretic underpinnings. *AJNR. American Journal of Neuroradiology*, 29 (4), 632–641.

Nucifora, P.G.P., *et al.*, 2005. Leftward asymmetry in relative fiber density of the arcuate fasciculus. *Neuroreport*, 16 (8), 791–794.

Ocklenburg, S., *et al.*, 2014. The ontogenesis of language lateralization and its relation to handedness. *Neuroscience and Biobehavioral Reviews*, 43, 191–198.

Ocklenburg, S., *et al.*, 2015. Laterality and mental disorders in the postgenomic age—A closer look at schizophrenia and language lateralization. *Neuroscience and Biobehavioral Reviews*, 59, 100–110.

Ocklenburg, S., *et al.*, 2016. Intrahemispheric white matter asymmetries: the missing link between brain structure and functional lateralization? *Reviews in the Neurosciences*, 27 (5), 465–480.

Ocklenburg, S., *et al.*, 2018. Neurite architecture of the planum temporale predicts neurophysiological processing of auditory speech. *Science Advances*, 4 (7), eaar6830.

Ocklenburg, S., and Güntürkün, O., 2018. *The lateralized brain. The neuroscience and evolution of hemispheric asymmetries.* London: Academic Press.

Ocklenburg, S., Hugdahl, K., and Westerhausen, R., 2013. Structural white matter asymmetries in relation to functional asymmetries during speech perception and production. *NeuroImage,* 83, 1088–1097.

Oertel-Knochel, V., *et al.*, 2012. Abnormal functional and structural asymmetry as biomarker for schizophrenia. *Current Topics in Medicinal Chemistry,* 12 (21), 2434–2451.

Oldfield, R.C., 1971. The assessment and analysis of handedness: the Edinburgh inventory. *Neuropsychologia,* 9 (1), 97–113.

Paracchini, S., Diaz, R., and Stein, J., 2016. Advances in Dyslexia genetics-new insights into the role of brain asymmetries. *Advances in Genetics,* 96, 53–97.

Pinel, P., and Dehaene, S., 2010. Beyond hemispheric dominance: brain regions underlying the joint lateralization of language and arithmetic to the left hemisphere. *Journal of Cognitive Neuroscience,* 22 (1), 48–66.

Reznik, S.J., and Allen, J.J.B., 2018. Frontal asymmetry as a mediator and moderator of emotion: an updated review. *Psychophysiology,* 55 (1).

Rogers, L.J., and Vallortigara, G., eds., 2017. *Lateralized brain functions. Methods in human and non-human species.* New York: Humana Press.

Savic, I., and Lindström, P., 2008. PET and MRI show differences in cerebral asymmetry and functional connectivity between homo- and heterosexual subjects. *Proceedings of the National Academy of Sciences of the United States of America,* 105 (27), 9403–9408.

Schmitz, J., *et al.*, 2017. Beyond the genome—towards an epigenetic understanding of handedness ontogenesis. *Progress in Neurobiology,* 159, 69–89.

Schmitz, J., *et al.*, 2019a. Hemispheric asymmetries in cortical gray matter microstructure identified by neurite orientation dispersion and density imaging. *NeuroImage,* 189, 667–675.

Schmitz, J., *et al.*, 2019b. Schizotypy and altered hemispheric asymmetries: the role of cilia genes. *Psychiatry Research. Neuroimaging,* 294, 110991.

Shapleske, J., *et al.*, 1999. The planum temporale: a systematic, quantitative review of its structural, functional and clinical significance. *Brain Research. Brain Research Reviews,* 29 (1), 26–49.

Smith, S.M., *et al.*, 2006. Tract-based spatial statistics: voxelwise analysis of multi-subject diffusion data. *NeuroImage,* 31 (4), 1487–1505.

Takao, H., Hayashi, N., and Ohtomo, K., 2011. White matter asymmetry in healthy individuals: a diffusion tensor imaging study using tract-based spatial statistics. *Neuroscience,* 193, 291–299.

Tervaniemi, M., and Hugdahl, K., 2003. Lateralization of auditory-cortex functions. *Brain Research. Brain Research Reviews,* 43 (3), 231–246.

Tournier, J.-D., and Mori, S., 2014. *Introduction to diffusion tensor imaging. And higher order models.* 2nd ed. Oxford, England and San Diego, CA: Academic Press.

Trinkl, M., *et al.*, 2015. Right-lateralization of N2-amplitudes in depressive adolescents: an emotional go/no-go study. *Journal of Child Psychology and Psychiatry, and Allied Disciplines,* 56 (1), 76–86.

Uomini, N.T., and Ruck, L., 2018. Manual laterality and cognition through evolution: an archeological perspective. *Progress in Brain Research*, 238, 295–323.

van der Haegen, L., *et al.*, 2013. Speech dominance is a better predictor of functional brain asymmetry than handedness: a combined fMRI word generation and behavioral dichotic listening study. *Neuropsychologia*, 51 (1), 91–97.

Veale, J.F., 2014. Edinburgh Handedness Inventory—Short form: a revised version based on confirmatory factor analysis. *Laterality*, 19 (2), 164–177.

Weir, K., 2012. The roots of mental illness. How much of mental illness can the biology of the brain explain? *Monitor on Psychology*, 43 (6), 30.

Westerhausen, R., *et al.*, 2015. Cognitive control of speech perception across the lifespan: a large-scale cross-sectional dichotic listening study. *Developmental Psychology*, 51 (6), 806–815.

Westerhausen, R., 2019. A primer on dichotic listening as a paradigm for the assessment of hemispheric asymmetry. *Laterality*, 24 (6), 740–771.

Westerhausen, R., and Kompus, K., 2018. How to get a left-ear advantage: a technical review of assessing brain asymmetry with dichotic listening. *Scandinavian Journal of Psychology*, 59 (1), 66–73.

WHO, 2016. International Classification of Disease-10. Available from: https://icd.who.int/browse10/2016/en.

Wildgruber, D., *et al.*, 2006. Cerebral processing of linguistic and emotional prosody: fMRI studies. *Progress in Brain Research*, 156, 249–268.

Zago, L., *et al.*, 2017. Pseudoneglect in line bisection judgement is associated with a modulation of right hemispheric spatial attention dominance in right-handers. *Neuropsychologia*, 94, 75–83.

Zahn, R., *et al.*, 2004. Hemispheric asymmetries of hypometabolism associated with semantic memory impairment in Alzheimer's disease: a study using positron emission tomography with fluorodeoxyglucose-F18. *Psychiatry Research*, 132 (2), 159–172.

Zhang, H., *et al.*, 2012. NODDI: practical in vivo neurite orientation dispersion and density imaging of the human brain. *NeuroImage*, 61 (4), 1000–1016.

Zhou, L., *et al.*, 2009. Detection of inter-hemispheric metabolic asymmetries in FDG-PET images using prior anatomical information. *NeuroImage*, 44 (1), 35–42.

Zhu, J., *et al.*, 2018. Abnormal gray matter asymmetry in alcohol dependence. *Neuroreport*, 29 (9), 753–759.

2 Lateralization in neurodevelopmental disorders

Introduction

Neurodevelopmental disorders are a class of disorders with onset during early development. Symptom manifestation usually begins before grade school. These disorders are characterized by developmental deficits compared to other children of the same age. They can lead to impairments in the emotional, social, personal, or academic life of the affected person. Different neurodevelopmental disorders frequently co-occur. Symptoms must persist for several months (approx. six months) to fulfil diagnostic criteria (American Psychiatric Association 2013).

Dyslexia

Definition of the disorder

Dyslexia is characterized by difficulties in reading despite normal intelligence (American Psychiatric Association 2013). Specifically, reading comprehension skills, reading word recognition, oral reading skills, and performance in tasks requiring reading may all be affected, mostly accompanied by spelling difficulties (WHO 2016). Dyslexia begins in early development and therefore is sometimes referred to as developmental dyslexia (WHO 2016). Irrespective of the country, an estimated 5–10% of the population is affected by dyslexia. The male to female ratio in epidemiological studies ranges from 1.5–3.3:1. One explanation might be greater variance in males' reading performance (Arnett *et al.* 2017). So far, there is no medical or neurobiological treatment for dyslexia even though the genetic and neuroanatomical alterations are quite well investigated. As yet, educational techniques that help the affected child to improve their reading skills are the only treatment option (Schulte-Körne 2010).

Theoretical models for the association between hemispheric asymmetries and dyslexia

Samuel Torrey Orton was the first scientist to suggest a link between atypical lateralization and developmental disorders (Orton 1937). He was especially interested in dyslexia and postulated that reading problems observed in dyslexia were actually caused by a failure to establish the left-right sense, which was caused by a failure to establish correct hemispheric dominance.

Several decades later, the probably most influential model regarding the association between hemispheric asymmetry and dyslexia was proposed. The Geschwind-Behan-Galaburda model (Geschwind and Behan 1982; Geschwind and Galaburda 1985a, 1985b, 1985c) assumes that testosterone plays a major role in linking developmental disorders to altered hemispheric asymmetries. Specifically, it is thought that high testosterone levels delay the maturation of the left hemisphere. Therefore, the right hemisphere is thought to play a greater role in various cognitive functions, like language, resulting in atypical lateralization patterns. Additionally, it is thought that high intrauterine testosterone levels negatively affect the development of left-temporal speech areas, resulting in a higher prevalence of dyslexia. The model has been criticized by several authors specifically because the link between testosterone and hemispheric asymmetries seems to be weaker than proposed (Berenbaum and Denburg 1995; Bryden *et al.* 1994; Previc 1994). The Geschwind-Behan-Galaburda model has been widely cited and is very influential in the field, providing important research impulses in clinical laterality research. However, substantial criticisms suggest that factors other than testosterone are more important for the association between dyslexia and atypical hemispheric asymmetries. Important theoretical contributions to clinical laterality research in the context of dyslexia research have also been made in terms of causality (Bishop 2013). These works will be discussed in Chapter 5 as they have more general relevance for the field that transcends specific theories about dyslexia.

Handedness

To date, two systematic investigations on the prevalence of non-right-handedness in dyslexia have been published. The first was conducted by Bishop (1990). Here, the author analysed 25 comparisons between individuals with dyslexia and healthy controls obtained from 21 individual studies. The analysis revealed an overall rate of left-handedness of 11.3% in individuals with dyslexia compared to 10.6% in healthy controls. This difference was not significant. The authors then conducted a second analysis in which the largest study was removed from the analysis since it might have had a disproportionately large impact on the overall result of the meta-analysis. In this analysis, there was an overall rate of left-handedness of 11.2% in individuals with dyslexia compared to 5.8% in healthy controls. This difference was significant, but it is striking that the effect seems to be driven by the fact that the healthy controls had a substantially lower rate of left-handedness than the 10.6% that has been observed in the general population (Papadatou-Pastou *et al.* 2020). Bishop (1990) concluded that the rate of left-handedness in dyslexia is well below what would be expected if atypical lateralization were indeed a cause of dyslexia.

Four years later, a meta-analysis on handedness in dyslexia reanalysing the dataset published in the book by Bishop (1990) was published (Eglinton and Annett 1994). Here, the authors used newer meta-analytic analysis techniques and found a small but reliable increase in the frequency of non-right-handedness in dyslexia. No exact percentages for the rate of non-right-handedness were given in the paper, but since the effect size was very small, the differences are unlikely to be large. Since both of these analyses are more than 25 years old by the time this book is written and their results are somewhat divergent, it would make sense to conduct a new meta-analysis on handedness in dyslexia to include primary research papers from the last 25 years.

Psychophysiological paradigms

Dyslexia is a developmental disorder of the language system. Therefore, it comes as no surprise that several studies have used psychophysical paradigms to investigate language lateralization in individuals with dyslexia on the behavioural level. Results were surprisingly mixed, suggesting a high heterogeneity in language lateralization in dyslexia (Obrzut and Boliek 1986). One early study using a divided visual field paradigm for word recognition reported typical leftward lateralization in adolescents with dyslexia (McKeever and VanDeventer 1975). Similarly, some studies did not report any differences between individuals with dyslexia and controls in language lateralization assessed with the dichotic listening task (Foster *et al.* 2002; Heiervang *et al.* 2000; Hakvoort *et al.* 2016), while others reported a reduced REA (right ear advantage) in dichotic listening in dyslexia (Hugdahl *et al.* 1995). Some authors have pointed out that symptom severity plays a crucial role in the association between dyslexia and altered language lateralization. One study of 125 boys reported that children with dyslexia showed lower absolute lateralization indices in a dichotic listening task, but that these differences only reached statistical significance when the most severe cases of dyslexia were analysed (Martínez and Sánchez 1999). A subgroup of children with mild dyslexia did not show any differences from controls.

A later study comparing dichotic listening performance in two groups of 12-year-old children with dyslexia, one with mild symptoms and one with more severe symptoms, also supported the idea that symptom severity is a crucial factor for the association between dyslexia and altered hemispheric asymmetries (Helland *et al.* 2008). Here, the children with mild symptoms showed REA comparable to controls, while the children with more severe dyslexia symptoms did not show REA. These findings highlight the importance of taking individual symptoms and not only diagnoses into account when assessing the relation of neurodevelopmental or psychiatric disorders and laterality, an idea that will be further elaborated in Chapter 5.

Functional hemispheric asymmetries in electrophysiological activity

While many studies have used EEG (electroencephalography) in individuals with dyslexia, it has not been used widely to specifically assess hemispheric asymmetries in this neurodevelopmental disorder. Similar to behavioural data, the EEG asymmetry data in dyslexia are rather heterogeneous. It has been reported that EEG alpha asymmetries during spontaneous speech do not differ between boys with dyslexia and normal-reading controls (Galin *et al.* 1988). A later study suggested that it is the theta band, but not the alpha band, which shows altered asymmetries in dyslexia (Spironelli *et al.* 2006). In this study, children with dyslexia were tested with a word-pair task with visual presentation. Compared to controls, they showed a rightward shift of theta activity but no significant differences in the alpha band. This finding was replicated in a later study with a similar task that also suggested a rightward shift of EEG beta asymmetries during linguistic tasks (Spironelli *et al.* 2008). For resting state EEG, a generally higher theta power in the left hemisphere in dyslexia has been reported (Papagiannopoulou and Lagopoulos 2016). It has also been suggested that mainly delta band asymmetries showed differences between individuals with dyslexia and controls with a more leftward anterior and a rightward posterior asymmetry in dyslexia (Penolazzi *et al.* 2008). In general, cohorts in these EEG asymmetry studies in dyslexia were small and larger studies are needed to clarify which of these effects replicate reliably.

Functional hemispheric asymmetries in brain activation

A substantial number of empirical studies on brain activation during language tasks have been published and some, but not all, suggest a reduction of the typical leftward brain activation asymmetry during language processing (De Guibert *et al.* 2011; Sun *et al.* 2010).

Several meta-analyses of neuroimaging studies have been published to assess systematic brain activation differences between individuals with dyslexia and controls. One early integration of neuroimaging studies of reading (Maisog *et al.* 2008) included two activation likelihood estimation (ALE) meta-analyses. The first included nine studies and identified brain regions in which typical readers showed significantly greater activations than individuals with dyslexia. This analysis identified nine clusters that showed differences between individuals and controls. Six of these clusters were in the left hemisphere (including language relevant areas, such as the inferior frontal gyrus) and three in the right hemisphere. The second analysis included six papers and was focused on regions in which individuals with dyslexia showed systematically greater brain activations than controls. This analysis revealed two right-hemispheric clusters (the right thalamus and anterior insula). This pattern of results led the authors to conclude that dyslexia is associated with greater right-hemispheric activity during reading.

One year later, an ALE meta-analysis of 17 neuroimaging studies with reading or reading-related tasks was published (Richlan *et al.* 2009). In this study, the authors reported that dyslexia was associated with a relative underactivation of several areas in the left hemisphere, including the superior, middle, and inferior temporal gyrus, the fusiform gyrus, and the inferior parietal gyrus. Thus, the findings of this study, in general, supported the findings of the earlier ALE in that they suggested a reduction of left-hemispheric brain activation during reading. A subsequent meta-analysis of 53 neuroimaging studies on language that was not restricted to reading tasks (Paulesu *et al.* 2014) reported similar results. In this study, the authors identified a network associated with reading in controls that showed reduced activation in individuals with dyslexia. This network included the left inferior frontal, premotor, and supramarginal cortices as well as the left inferotemporal and fusiform brain regions.

Most recently, an ALE meta-analysis of 13 cross-linguistic neuroimaging studies on reading (Pollack *et al.* 2015) compared brain activation during reading in typical readers and atypical readers, which included individuals with dyslexia, but also subclinical groups with reading difficulties. In this study, the authors reported that typical readers showed significant activations only in the left hemisphere, specifically in the inferior frontal gyrus, the precentral gyrus, and the middle temporal gyrus. Atypical readers additionally showed activations in the left inferior frontal area and precentral region, several right-hemispheric regions in the frontal and occipital lobe.

Taken together, the evidence from meta-analyses of neuroimaging studies consistently suggests a reduction of leftward language asymmetries during reading in dyslexia.

Structural hemispheric asymmetries in grey matter

The planum temporale (PT) is one of the most asymmetric grey matter structures in the human brain, showing a pronounced leftward asymmetry in healthy individuals. While several early studies have reported reduced structural hemispheric asymmetries in the PT in dyslexia, there were also several studies not supporting this association (Beaton 1997). Early descriptive integration of neuroimaging studies (Shapleske *et al.* 1999) reported that, out of eight studies measuring PT asymmetry in dyslexia, four reported symmetry or reduced asymmetry of the PT due to smaller left plana in dyslexia. One study reported reduced asymmetry due to the larger right plana. Based on these findings, Shapleske *et al.* (1999) suggested that dyslexia may be associated with reduced asymmetry of the PT.

A meta-analytic integration of nine voxel-based morphometry studies that investigated local grey matter differences between individuals with dyslexia and controls (Linkersdörfer *et al.* 2012) reported six clusters of significant convergence between the included studies, of which all six showed relative reductions of grey matter. The largest cluster was observed in the left fusiform gyrus extending into the left inferior temporal gyrus, followed by clusters in the left supramarginal gyrus and the left cerebellum. In the right hemisphere, reductions were also found in the supramarginal gyrus and the cerebellum but to a lesser extent than in the left hemisphere. Additionally, a cluster in the right superior temporal gyrus was reported. A few years later, a signed differential mapping meta-analysis of eleven voxel-based morphometry studies (Eckert *et al.* 2016) reported that dyslexia was associated with lower grey matter volumes in the left posterior superior temporal sulcus, middle temporal gyrus, and left orbitofrontal gyrus (pars orbitalis). Taken together, these findings suggest that dyslexia is associated with a loss of grey matter volume in left-hemispheric frontotemporal networks associated with reading and language processing in general.

Structural hemispheric asymmetries in white matter

A substantial amount of neuroimaging studies have investigated white matter structure in dyslexia and in 2012, a meta-analysis of nine diffusion tensor imaging (DTI) studies in individuals with dyslexia was published (Vandermosten *et al.* 2012). The authors found that one large cluster, located close to the left temporoparietal region, showed reduced fractional anisotropy in individuals with dyslexia. Further analysis revealed that this cluster likely included fibres belonging to the left arcuate fasciculus and the left corona radiata, two fibre tracts that had previously been shown to be relevant for reading. A study in adults with dyslexia confirmed reduced leftward asymmetry of the arcuate fasciculus (Vandermosten *et al.* 2013), while a subsequent study in French children with dyslexia and age-matched controls reported reduced leftward lateralization of the inferior fronto-occipital fasciculus, as well as increased rightward asymmetry of the second branch of the superior longitudinal fasciculus, but no group difference for the arcuate fasciculus (Zhao *et al.* 2016). A subsequent study, however, again showed evidence for a reduced leftward asymmetry of the arcuate fasciculus in dyslexia (Banfi *et al.* 2019).

Taken together, an updated meta-analytical integration of neuroimaging studies on white matter asymmetries in dyslexia would be needed to resolve these slight inconsistencies. However, based on the 2012 meta-analysis and two subsequent studies, a reduced leftward asymmetry of the arcuate fasciculus seems to be the most reliably altered aspect of structural white matter asymmetries in dyslexia. Since the arcuate fasciculus is an important white matter tract in the language system, connecting Wernicke's area to Broca's area among others, this finding is in line with the general idea of a more right-hemispheric organization of language networks in dyslexia.

Genetics

Hemispheric asymmetries and dyslexia seem to show some genetic overlap. In an influential review article, Brandler and Paracchini (2014) suggested that cilia might be a factor that links dyslexia and hemispheric asymmetries. Cilia are cell organelles that play a key role in establishing bodily left-right asymmetries during development. Empirical evidence links cilia to both dyslexia and hemispheric asymmetries. For example, increased expression of *DCDC2*, a dyslexia susceptibility gene, affects both length and signalling of cilia in neurons (Massinen *et al.* 2011). Moreover, comparative research in zebrafish has suggested that the zebrafish orthologue of *DYX1C1*, another dyslexia susceptibility gene, plays a central role in cilia growth and function (Chandrasekar *et al.* 2013). It has also been suggested that *PCSK6*, a gene that is functionally relevant for bodily left-right asymmetries, provides a link between dyslexia and handedness. A relation of *PCSK6* and handedness had first been reported in a dyslexic cohort (Scerri *et al.* 2011) but was later also reported in candidate gene studies in non-dyslexic cohorts (Arning *et al.* 2013; Robinson *et al.* 2016). Besides, it has been shown that methylation of the promotor region of *KIAA0319*, a gene that had been related to both ciliogenesis and dyslexia, predicts dichotic listening performance (Schmitz *et al.* 2018). Altogether, the idea that cilia provide a link between dyslexia and hemispheric asymmetries is an interesting hypothesis and future studies in larger cohorts should further investigate this assumption.

Conclusion

Taken together, there is substantial evidence for less leftward language lateralization in dyslexia both on the functional as well as on the structural level. Several meta-analyses of functional neuroimaging studies mostly related to reading suggested reduced leftward brain activation in functional language networks. These altered functional asymmetries in the language network were mirrored by less leftward structural asymmetries in the grey matter as well as reduced leftward lateralization of the arcuate fasciculus, the major white matter tract in the language system. Research on the behavioural level was less unequivocal, but instead highlighted the importance of taking symptom severity into account when assessing altered hemispheric asymmetries in neurodevelopmental disorders. Genetic studies suggest a role of cilia in connecting dyslexia and altered hemispheric asymmetries, but more research is needed in this field.

Attention deficit hyperactivity disorder

Definition of the disorder

Another neurodevelopmental disorder that has been associated with atypical hemispheric lateralization is attention deficit hyperactivity disorder (ADHD). It was first described in 1775 by the German doctor Melchior Adam Weikard as a disorder with "a lack of attention" (Weikard 1775–77). Nowadays, ADHD is defined by interfering inattention and/or hyperactivity-impulsivity of the child leading to impaired functioning (American Psychiatric Association 2013). The disorder is characterized by three main symptoms: being overactive, having difficulties in paying attention, and acting without prior thinking thus being impulsive. Which of these symptoms is most prominent varies throughout development (American Psychiatric Association 2013). As a neurodevelopmental disorder, ADHD typically begins in childhood but can persist into adulthood. Worldwide, around 5% of children and 2.5% of adults are affected (American Psychiatric Association 2013). Men are more than twice as likely to be affected than women (Ramtekkar *et al.* 2010).

ADHD has a highly heritable component which points to a genetic aetiology (Burt 2009). Twin studies including family members, such as siblings and cousins, analysing the occurrence of ADHD underlined the role of a genetic factor (Chen *et al.* 2017). In a genome-wide association study (GWAS), multiple risk loci on different chromosomes have been linked to ADHD with many of the implied genes playing a role in brain plasticity (Demontis *et al.* 2019). Environmental influences seem to play a less important role (Burt 2009). However, substance use during pregnancy, perinatal nutritional factors, and heavy metal and chemical exposure have been associated with an increased risk for ADHD (Froehlich *et al.* 2011). Behavioural therapy, such as conditioning to reinforce desirable behaviour and behavioural parent training, is highly effective for treating ADHD symptoms (Fabiano *et al.* 2009). Most effective is a combined treatment with psychotherapy and pharmacotherapy (Wigal 2009). In terms of pharmacotherapy, the use of amphetamine-based or methylphenidate-based stimulants is most successful (Wigal 2009).

The right-hemisphere deficit hypothesis of ADHD

Having difficulties paying attention is one of the core symptoms of ADHD as described previously and there is substantial evidence suggesting a right-hemispheric dominance for visuospatial attention (Bowers and Heilman 1980; Heilman *et al.* 1986; Heilman and van den Abell 1980). Moreover, patients with right-hemispheric lesions or dysfunction more often show attentional deficits than patients with left-hemispheric lesions or dysfunctions (Heilman *et al.* 1991; Klimkeit and Bradshaw 2006; Stefanatos and Wasserstein 2001). Based on these findings, it has been suggested that ADHD represents a specific dysfunction of the right hemisphere (Heilman *et al.* 1991), an idea that has been hugely influential for subsequent studies.

Handedness

Meta-analysis (Nastou *et al.* 2020) indicated that ADHD was associated with a higher prevalence of mixed-handedness (15.19% in ADHD, 9.33% in controls). For left-handedness and non-right-handedness, no group differences were observed. Moreover, it has been shown that mixed-handers show higher inattentiveness than left- or right-handers, while no differences were found for hyperactivity and impulsivity (Lin and Tsuang 2018). Furthermore, a large internet study with 255,100 subjects reported that people with mixed preferences for writing hand had a significantly higher prevalence of hyperactivity than people with a clear left- or right-hand preference for writing (Peters *et al.* 2006).

Psychophysiological paradigms

An early dichotic listening study found that both hyperactive children and healthy controls showed a similar REA for verbal stimuli (Davidson and Prior 1978). Similar results were also observed by more recent dichotic listening studies in children (Foster *et al.* 2002) and adults (Dramsdahl *et al.* 2011; Hale *et al.* 2006). Thus, the empirical evidence suggests that language lateralization is not altered in ADHD. As language is processed by the left hemisphere in most individuals, this result is in line with the idea that ADHD is mostly affecting brain areas in the right hemisphere. Also, in addition to studies with verbal dichotic listening tasks, one study used a dichotic listening task with emotional stimuli (Hale *et al.* 2006). In this study, patients also showed a typical pattern (left ear advantage, LEA) comparable to healthy controls. A study using a divided visual field paradigm for metaphor processing found that controls showed a left visual field/right hemisphere dominance that was reduced in ADHD patients (Segal *et al.* 2017), supported the idea of a specific right hemisphere deficit in ADHD.

To test the idea of a right hemispheric deficit in ADHD, several studies have used the line bisection task (Jewell and McCourt 2000). Results obtained with the task have been rather heterogeneous. While one early study reported that ADHD was associated with further rightward line bisection than in healthy controls (Sheppard *et al.* 1999), later studies reported unaltered pseudoneglect in ADHD in the line bisection task (Helfer *et al.* 2020) and other behavioural measures of visuospatial attention (Klimkeit *et al.* 2003). Further research has suggested that specifically right-hemispheric tasks that require interhemispheric networking are affected in ADHD and not right-hemispheric tasks per se (Hale *et al.* 2009b). Moreover, it has been reported that only the combined subtype of ADHD but not the predominantly inattentive subtype of ADHD shows a right-hemisphere deficit (Rolfe *et al.* 2006). Taken together, the behavioural evidence does not unequivocally support the idea of a general right-hemispheric deficit in ADHD.

Functional hemispheric asymmetries in electrophysiological activity

Increased rightward EEG alpha asymmetries have been reported for adults with ADHD (Hale *et al.* 2009a), indicating reduced right-hemispheric activation. Similar results have also been reported for boys with ADHD, while girls with ADHD showed the opposite pattern (Baving *et al.* 1999). A more recent study in adolescents reported that a rightward EEG alpha asymmetry was only present in those individuals with ADHD who showed low levels of negative affect (Alperin *et al.* 2019). Moreover, a pronounced rightward asymmetry in parietal EEG beta asymmetries has been reported in adults with ADHD (Hale *et al.* 2010) and was also replicated in a subsequent study (Hale *et al.* 2014). As EEG beta is thought to reflect cognitive activity, these findings suggest an increased rather than decreased right-hemispheric activation in the parietal lobe, arguing against the right-hemisphere deficit model.

Functional hemispheric asymmetries in brain activation

One ALE meta-analysis of 16 functional neuroimaging studies mostly focused on response inhibition (Dickstein *et al.* 2006) and reported that ADHD patients had significantly higher activation probabilities for two left frontal areas, the left insular cortex, and parts of the left middle frontal gyrus. Moreover, increased activation in ADHD was observed in the left thalamus and the right paracentral lobule, and ADHD patients had significantly lower activation probabilities than controls for the left dorsal and ventral prefrontal cortex, the anterior cingulate cortex, both the left and the right parietal lobe, the right thalamus, the left middle occipital gyrus, and the right claustrum. Thus, while the increased activations in individuals with ADHD somewhat support a more left-hemispheric mode of processing, the deactivations do not follow any hemisphere specific pattern and seem to be rather region-specific.

More than a decade later, a substantially larger neuroimaging meta-analysis of 96 ADHD studies reported no significant clusters that show systematic alteration of asymmetry between individuals with ADHD and controls (Samea *et al.* 2019). A sub-analysis in which only fMRI studies with neutral stimuli were included showed that individuals with ADHD showed aberrant activity in the left pallidum and putamen. Moreover, in male ADHD subjects only, decreased activity was observed in the left inferior frontal gyrus. While the finding of aberrant activity in the left basal ganglia in this one specific analysis might support the right-hemisphere deficit model of ADHD to some extent, the lack of any effects in the overall analysis suggests that there is no general rightward shift of brain activations in ADHD.

Structural hemispheric asymmetries in grey matter

Several studies have investigated structural grey matter asymmetries in ADHD, mostly focusing on the basal ganglia and frontal areas due to their involvement in attentional processes. One frequently reported finding is a left-shift in basal ganglia asymmetries in ADHD, potentially reflecting a deficit of the right hemisphere (Paclt *et al.* 2016). For example, one early study reported a rightward asymmetry of caudate nucleus volume in typically developing controls that was absent in ADHD (Castellanos *et al.* 1994). This finding was reported by a subsequent study, which also reported a smaller right globus pallidus and a smaller right anterior frontal region in ADHD (Castellanos *et al.* 1996). A later study reported a leftward asymmetry for globus pallidus and caudate nucleus in ADHD (Uhlíková *et al.* 2007). Structural hemispheric asymmetries in the basal ganglia have also been associated with ADHD symptom severity. For example, one study reported that the degree of hemispheric asymmetry in the caudate significantly predicted the severity of inattentive behaviours (Schrimsher *et al.* 2002). Later, it was reported that larger rightward volume asymmetry in the caudate correlated with higher attentional impulsiveness and worse ADHD scores (Dang *et al.* 2016).

In addition to altered basal ganglia asymmetries, changes in frontal asymmetries have been reported in ADHD. One developmental study in 218 children with ADHD and 358 controls reported that typically developing children showed a right-left asymmetry in the increase of the relative thickness of the orbitofrontal and inferior frontal cortex during development. This asymmetry was absent in ADHD (Shaw *et al.* 2009). However, on the meta-analytical level, basal ganglia asymmetry alterations seem to be more stable than frontal asymmetry alterations. One meta-analysis of only seven neuroimaging studies with an overall sample size of 114 patients with ADHD or related disorders and 143 controls reported and significant grey matter reduction in the right putamen/globus pallidus of ADHD patients (Ellison-Wright *et al.* 2008).

Interestingly, the largest published study on grey matter asymmetries in ADHD is somewhat at odds with the previously published literature. In this study (Douglas *et al.* 2018), the authors obtained structural MRI scans from 341 children and adolescents with ADHD and 508 neurotypical controls and determined volumetric asymmetries in 34 cortical and 14 non-cortical brain regions. The authors reported that there were no significant differences in the asymmetry index of any investigated brain region when comparing medication-free individuals with ADHD to typically developing individuals. However, the absolute asymmetry index, indicating the strength of lateralization independently of its direction, showed significant differences between the two groups for eleven cortical brain regions, mainly centred around cingulate and parietal regions. Importantly, the magnitude of the asymmetry index was increased in individuals with ADHD compared to typically developing controls for all eleven brain regions. This indicates increased structural asymmetries in grey matter in ADHD on an individual level, without a general shift to one hemisphere on the population level as previous studies suggested. For subcortical regions, similar results were also observed for the amygdala but not the basal ganglia. Moreover, the authors conducted a morphometric analysis to assess the detailed shape of subcortical nuclei. In this analysis, they found that caudate, hippocampus, thalamus, and amygdala showed greater morphometric asymmetries in ADHD individuals compared to typically developing controls. The finding of an increased asymmetry in the caudate is more in line with the previously published literature than the volumetric analysis, while the other results suggest that structural asymmetry changes in ADHD are not limited to the basal ganglia but also affect other subcortical structures.

Structural hemispheric asymmetries in white matter

In addition to altered grey matter asymmetries, a few recent studies have reported altered white matter asymmetries in ADHD. For example, typically developing individuals show a rightward connectivity asymmetry between the caudate nucleus and the dorsolateral prefrontal cortex and the ventrolateral prefrontal cortex (Silk *et al.* 2016). This rightward asymmetry was absent in individuals with ADHD. This is in line with the findings for grey matter structural asymmetries, suggesting that mostly networks involving prefrontal areas and the basal ganglia show altered asymmetries in ADHD. In 104 subjects, Douglas *et al.* (2018) found group differences in asymmetry indices for DTI mean diffusivity for the cingulum as well as for the inferior and superior longitudinal fasciculus and cortico-spinal tracts. Both the comparison for the asymmetry indices and the absolute asymmetry indices reached significance indicating larger and more leftward asymmetries in ADHD for most tracts. The most recent study reported an increased leftward asymmetry of the posterior thalamic radiation in ADHD, a tract that had not been previously associated with ADHD (Wu *et al.* 2020). In addition to these tract-based studies, a graph theory-based study reported that ADHD was associated with reduced asymmetries in global and local network integration (Li *et al.* 2019). In particular, controls showed a rightward asymmetry for global network efficiency that was notably absent in ADHD. Altogether, the literature on white matter asymmetries in ADHD is inconclusive, and additional analyses in larger cohorts are needed before any final conclusions can be drawn.

Genetics

Only few studies have investigated the genetic overlap between ADHD and hemispheric asymmetries. One study investigated the association of genetic variation in six genes that had shown substantial expression asymmetries in a previous study (at least 1.9-fold differential expression between the two hemispheres) with ADHD (Ribasés *et al.* 2009). In a sample of 587 ADHD patients and 587 controls, the authors found a significant association of genetic variation in *BAIAP2* and ADHD. This finding replicated in a German control sample but not in a Norwegian control sample. A later study also suggested that genetic variation in *BAIAP2* was related to both connectivity asymmetry of the medial frontal gyrus and inferior parietal lobule and externalization of anger in ADHD (Hasler *et al.* 2017). This suggests that *BAIAP2* might be a potential genetic link between ADHD and hemispheric asymmetries, but replication studies are needed.

More recently, a large-scale GWAS using the UK Biobank dataset (n=18,057) reported that two single nucleotide polymorphisms (rs41298373 and rs7420166) showed a significant association with PT volume asymmetry (Carrion-Castillo *et al.* 2020). However, no significant genetic correlations of PT asymmetry and ADHD were observed, arguing for little to no overlap of the genetic determinants of this specific structural asymmetry and those of ADHD. In general, further large-scale studies focusing on different asymmetry phenotypes and their genetic overlap with ADHD are needed before any final conclusions can be drawn.

Conclusion

Taken together, ADHD presents an interesting case in clinical laterality research. The handedness data suggest a link between mixed-handedness and ADHD. In general, the right-hemisphere deficit hypothesis has been highly influential in the ADHD laterality literature, but empirical evidence from behavioural studies, EEG data, and neuroimaging meta-analysis do not yield strong support for this model, although there is some supporting evidence. On the structural level, early studies consistently suggested stronger leftward asymmetries of the basal ganglia, but a newer large-scale study suggested the strength of structural grey matter asymmetries is higher in ADHD without a specific direction effect. This is highly unusual as, in most other neurodevelopmental and psychiatric disorders, structural asymmetries are reduced rather than increased. Therefore, this finding clearly deserves more investigation. No clear pattern emerged for white matter asymmetries.

Autism spectrum disorders

Definition of the disorder

Another group of developmental disorders associated with atypical lateralization is autism spectrum disorder (ASD). In the 1940s, Leo Kanner published his description of children suffering from a disorder he termed autism. Back then, he noticed that these children were unable to relate to others, showed social withdrawal, repetitive behaviour, and unusual language development (Kanner 1943). Around the same time, Hans Asperger published his findings of children with similar psychopathology with primary problems in non-verbal communication and social skills (Asperger 1944).

ASD is characterized by persistent impairment in reciprocal social communication and interaction, nonverbal and verbal communication, and restricted, stereotyped, repetitive behaviour or interests. Moreover, children suffering from ASD show deficits in social-emotional reciprocity, in nonverbal communicative behaviours used for social interaction, and in developing, maintaining, and understanding relationships. Symptoms begin in early childhood. ASD affects around 1% of the general population with men being affected four times more frequently than women (Werling and Geschwind 2013; American Psychiatric Association 2013).

Several studies have investigated the genetic basis of ASD. The results suggest that deletions or duplications of nucleotides in the DNA sequence or copy number variations of specific genes, whether they are inherited or occur *de novo*, increase the risk of ASD (Masi *et al.* 2017). Environmental factors, such as maternal infection during pregnancy (Patterson 2011) or an advanced paternal age, may also be responsible for developing ASD. But as for most psychiatric disorders, a gene-environment interaction is postulated (Chaste and Leboyer 2012). So far, there is no pharmacological treatment available to treat the core symptoms of ASD. Thus, the gold standard is behavioural intervention, if possible, early in life, to treat the behavioural symptoms and to provide strategies for social interactions. New studies investigate whether treatment with oxytocin might be helpful to improve social-cognitive functions (Hohagen and Voderholzer 2019).

Handedness

Several studies systematically reviewing or meta-analysing handedness in ASD have been published (Lindell and Hudry 2013; Markou *et al.* 2017; Preslar *et al.* 2014; Rysstad and Pedersen 2016). In the latest meta-analysis, the authors revealed a significantly elevated rate of atypical handedness in individuals with ASD (N=723) compared to healthy controls (N=476). More precisely, they found that the general prevalence of non-right-handedness in ASD is 45.4%, the prevalence of left-handedness is 18.3% and the prevalence of mixed-handedness is 36.1% (left-handedness and mixed-handedness combined resulted in a higher percentage than that observed for non-right-handedness as different studies were included in the different analyses) (Markou *et al.* 2017). This is one of the most substantial increases in non-right-handedness observed for any neurodevelopmental or psychiatric disorder.

Psychophysiological paradigms

Markou *et al.* (2017) suggested that the increased rate of non-right-handedness in individuals with ASD might be linked to atypical language lateralization. The question of whether language lateralization is altered in ASD has been investigated in several behavioural studies (Lindell and Hudry 2013). Three early verbal dichotic listening studies reported a decrease of the typically observed right ear advantage (REA) in this task, indicating a stronger role of right-hemispheric networks for language processing in ASD than in typically developing individuals (Blackstock 1978; Prior and Bradshaw 1979; Hayashi *et al.* 1989). This alteration of functional lateralization in dichotic listening seems to be specific for the language domain, as a study using an emotional dichotic listening paradigm did not observe any significant difference between individuals with ASD and typically developing controls (Baker *et al.* 2010).

Interestingly, the reduction or reversal of typical functional hemispheric asymmetries for language processing in ASD is not limited to left-hemispheric language functions. In a divided visual field paradigm, control participants (*N*=36) showed a right-hemispheric superiority for metaphor processing, while ASD participants (*N*=27) did not show a hemispheric asymmetry (Gold and Faust 2010). This suggests that ASD might be related to reduced functional lateralization in the language domain in general, rather than a specific rightward shift.

Reduced functional lateralization in ASD is also found in cognitive domains other than language. For example, a study on hemispheric asymmetries in visuospatial attention reported a reduced pseudoneglect (the typical leftward attentional bias observed in neurotypical individuals) in ASD, suggesting reduced functional hemispheric asymmetries for visuospatial attention in ASD (English *et al.* 2017).

Functional hemispheric asymmetries in electrophysiological activity

A small number of EEG studies have investigated altered hemispheric asymmetries in ASD. One early study compared EEG alpha asymmetries in 21 children with ASD and 28 healthy controls (Ogawa *et al.* 1982). The authors reported that significant lateralization was observed only in controls but not in children with ASD. A later study focused on the development of frontal EEG alpha asymmetry in 57 infants with a high risk to develop ASD and 51 infants with a low risk to develop ASD (Gabard-Durnam *et al.* 2015). At 6 months of age, low-risk infants showed significant right frontal asymmetry, while the asymmetry score in high-risk infants did not differ significantly from zero. This indicated no hemispheric asymmetry in frontal EEG alpha activity in the high-risk group which is in line with the findings of the earlier study by Ogawa *et al.* (1982). Thus, both studies suggest reduced frontal alpha asymmetries in ASD.

Functional hemispheric asymmetries in brain activation

Recently, 22 published fMRI and PET studies using different language tasks like semantic processing, sentence comprehension, or speech production were integrated into an ALE meta-analysis (Herringshaw *et al.* 2016). Overall, 328 individuals with ASD and 324 controls were included. While language-related activation largely overlapped between the ASD group and the control group, the authors observed several differences in hemispheric asymmetries between the two groups. Most importantly, the ASD group showed more rightward activity in core language areas such as the superior temporal gyrus and the inferior frontal gyrus compared to controls. Additionally, the ASD group showed a bilateral hypoactivation in the middle temporal gyrus and increased activation in the left lingual gyrus compared to controls. Thus, individuals with ASD seem to process language to a larger extent in the right hemisphere than typically developing controls. The authors suggest that the increased activation in the left lingual gyrus, a brain area that has been associated with reading, might reflect compensatory processes. Interestingly, an fMRI study published a few years later found that reduced language lateralization due to higher right hemisphere activity was also associated with autistic traits (N=189) (Jouravlev *et al.* 2020).

A rightward shift in functional brain activation in ASD was not only reported for language-related functional tasks, but also resting-state connectivity in a wide variety of functional networks, including language networks, but also visual, auditory, motor, executive, and attentional networks (Cardinale *et al.* 2013). This indicates that a more rightward organization of functional networks might be a feature of brain organization in ASD that extends beyond language networks.

Structural hemispheric asymmetry in grey matter

While some studies did not observe any differences in structural asymmetries of grey matter regions between individuals with ASD and controls (Joseph *et al.* 2014; Knaus *et al.* 2012; Preslar *et al.* 2014), others reported significant differences in varying brain regions (Dougherty *et al.* 2016; Floris *et al.* 2016; Fu *et al.* 2020).

The largest study on alterations in structural hemispheric asymmetries in grey matter in ASD was conducted by the ENIGMA consortium (Postema *et al.* 2019). The authors investigated asymmetries in thickness and surface area measures for 34 cortical regions and 7 subcortical regions in a dataset consisting of 1774 individuals with ASD and 1809 controls from 54 independent data sets. After correction for multiple comparisons, ten effects reached significance. For thickness asymmetry, seven regions showed significant differences between individuals with ASD and controls. These included areas in the frontal lobe (superior frontal, rostral middle frontal, medial orbitofrontal), areas in the temporal lobe (fusiform, inferior temporal) as well as cingulate areas (rostral anterior, isthmus cingulate). For surface asymmetry, three regions reached significance, including the medial- and lateral orbitofrontal cortex and the putamen. For all observed effects, effect sizes were low (Cohen's d between -0.13 and 0.12), indicating subtle rather than substantial changes in structural grey matter asymmetries in ASD. This also highlights the need for large samples with high statistical power to detect such changes reliably and implies that many previous studies on this topic were underpowered. For all cortical regions, individuals with ASD showed reduced hemispheric asymmetries, no matter whether the region on average showed a left-hemispheric or right-hemispheric asymmetry. Out of the nine significant regions, six showed a decrease of leftward asymmetries and three a decrease of rightward asymmetries. Thus, ASD seems to be related to a general reduction in cortical asymmetries, not a shift in one or the other direction. For the putamen, individuals with ASD interestingly showed an increased rightward asymmetry compared to controls. The authors point out that some of the brain areas showing altered hemispheric asymmetries in ASD have been linked to social-cognitive processes such as emotional control and reward evaluation, but that there were also altered hemispheric asymmetries in brain areas unrelated to the symptoms commonly associated with ASD. Therefore, they argue that ASD is linked to a broad disruption of lateralized neurodevelopment, rather than a specific disruption of ASD-associated cognitive systems.

Structural hemispheric asymmetries in white matter

Many studies on structural white matter asymmetries in ASD report a reduction or reversal of structural asymmetries observed in neurotypical individuals. For example, it has been reported that typically developing individuals show an overall rightward asymmetry of fractional anisotropy, a marker of structural integrity of white matter. This asymmetry is reduced in ASD (Carper *et al.* 2016). Reduced or reversed structural hemispheric asymmetries have also been reported on the level of specific tracts. For example, one study in five completely nonverbal children with ASD found that they did not show the typical leftward asymmetry of the arcuate fasciculus, a major white matter tract in the language system (Wan *et al.* 2012). Instead, four out of five children showed an inverted rightward asymmetry in this tract. A later study in 20 children with ASD and 20 typically developing controls also reported a reduced leftward asymmetry in the arcuate fasciculus (Joseph *et al.* 2014). Reversed structural white matter asymmetries in ASD have also been reported for the white matter underlying the superior temporal gyrus (Lange *et al.* 2010). A meta-analysis of 14 DTI studies in ASD and controls that were not specifically targeted at hemispheric asymmetries (Aoki *et al.* 2013) reported that individuals with ASD showed significant reductions of fractional anisotropy in clusters in the corpus callosum, the left uncinate fasciculus, and the left superior longitudinal fasciculus, indicating an underconnectivity in the left hemisphere of individuals with ASD.

Importantly, a recent High-Angular-Resolution Diffusion Imaging protocol (HARDI) diffusion MRI study (Conti *et al.* 2016) reported evidence for significant associations between lateralization of various white matter diffusion indices for frontotemporal tracts and clinical severity of ASD in a sample of 20 children (36 months or younger) with ASD. Importantly, all correlations were negative, indicating that children with higher clinical severity of ASD were more likely to show reversed structural asymmetries in frontotemporal circuits relevant for socio-communicative skills.

Comparative research

Hemispheric asymmetries have not been a major focus in comparative studies on ASD. One study (Grabrucker *et al.* 2017) reported that prenatal zinc-deficient mice, a mouse model with ASD-like behaviour, exhibit altered hemispheric asymmetries. Specifically, the authors reported that control mice showed expression asymmetries in several genes (*Arrb2*, *Gap43*, *Neurod6*, *Pclo*, and *Pkcβ*) that were not found in the ASD model. Moreover, the ASD model mice showed reduced side preferences in turning behaviour tests. Thus, the results of this study suggest the ASD model mice show reduced lateralization on several levels, which is in line with the results of some of the aforementioned studies in human subjects.

Genetics

Very few studies explicitly investigated the overlap in genetic factors relevant to hemispheric asymmetries and ASD. One candidate gene study in 709 healthy subjects (Robinson *et al.* 2016) found that genetic variation in

PCSK6, a gene that had previously been linked to handedness and plays a role in left-right axis determination during embryogenesis (Scerri *et al.* 2011), was associated with both handedness and autistic traits. However, since no individuals with an actual ASD diagnosis were included in this study, it is unclear to what extent these findings apply to ASD. Moreover, the same large-scale GWAS using the UK Biobank dataset (Carrion-Castillo *et al.* 2020), also reported no significant genetic correlation of PT asymmetry and ASD, arguing for little to no overlap of the genetic determinants of this specific structural asymmetry and genetic factors associated with ASD. In general, further large-scale studies focusing on different asymmetry phenotypes and their genetic overlap with ASD are needed before any final conclusions can be drawn.

Conclusion

Taken together, there is robust evidence for altered hemispheric asymmetries on many levels in ASD. ASD is related to a substantial increase in non-right-handedness, as well as a reduction of the typical leftward asymmetry in language processing as evidenced by behavioural, EEG, and neuroimaging studies. Moreover, several grey and white matter studies revealed reduced structural asymmetries in individuals with ASD compared to neurotypical controls. While the genetic links between hemispheric asymmetries and ASD remain largely unclear, these findings suggest that a reduction of hemispheric asymmetries is an integral part of the neurobiology of ASD.

Stuttering

Definition of the disorder

Stuttering is a disorder in which the normal fluency and time patterning of speech is disrupted (American Psychiatric Association 2013). The onset of symptoms is during early development, ranging from two to seven years of age, and is marked by disturbances that do not match the individual's age, marked by sound and syllable repetition, prolongation of consonants, pauses or hesitations within a word or during speech (American Psychiatric Association 2013). Around 70–80% of children recover from stuttering, but the disorder can also persist into adolescence and adulthood with around 1% of children and adolescents and 0.2% of women and 0.8% of men suffering from the disorder (Neumann *et al.* 2017).

So far, no environmental influence on the development of stuttering is known, but a high heritability (69–85%) of the disorder has been observed

(Neumann *et al.* 2017). First-degree biological relatives of people suffering from stuttering show three times increased risk for the development of the disorder (Kraft and Yairi 2012; Neumann *et al.* 2017). Different studies investigating stuttering in various countries found specific genetic loci on multiple chromosomes which were associated with an increased risk for stuttering (Kraft and Yairi 2012). However, each study revealed different chromosomes being affected. Some researchers argue that dopamine signalling might be disrupted in stuttering. Thus, when investigating the variation in two dopaminergic genes and stuttering in a Chinese population, a specific single nucleotide polymorphism in the *DRD2* gene was found to increase the risk to develop the disorder (Chen *et al.* 2014). As no medical treatment is known to lower the symptoms, the main symptoms are treated mainly with speech training from early on (Neumann *et al.* 2017).

Handedness

In 1947, one of the first scientists to link stuttering and atypical hemispheric lateralization by investigating handedness in stuttering children was Kypros Chrysanthis. He reported a more than fourfold increase in left-handedness in children suffering from stuttering (Chrysanthis 1947). However, later studies in larger samples could not replicate this finding. For example, one study from 1987 compared stuttering in 241 left-handers and 178 right-handers (van Strien *et al.* 1987). The authors found that 6.2% of left-handers and 6.1% of right-handers stuttered, a difference that failed to reach significance. Similarly, a study that compared handedness prevalence between adults who stuttered and non-stuttering controls found no significant differences between the two groups (Webster and Poulos 1987). Altogether, the empirical evidence suggests that there is no association between stuttering and left-handedness. Historically, it has also been assumed that stuttering is not related to left-handedness per se, but to forcing left-handers to write with their right hand (Kushner 2012). Retraining was thought to lead to a confusion of cerebral dominance which in turn resulted in stuttering.

Psychophysiological paradigms

As stuttering is a speech disorder, it comes as no surprise that several researchers have used the dichotic listening task to investigate language lateralization in individuals who stutter. An early study from the 1960s compared dichotic listening performance in 20 individuals who stutter and 20 controls (Curry and Gregory 1969). In this study, the researchers reported that most controls (75%) showed a REA, while most individuals who stutter showed an LEA (55%). However, subsequent studies yielded highly ambiguous results with some studies supporting the idea of a reduced REA or even LEA in individuals who stutter (Sommers *et al.* 1975; Strub *et al.* 1987). However, a larger amount of studies reported no significant differences between individuals who stutter and controls in language lateralization assessed with the dichotic listening task (Dorman and Porter 1975; Gruber and Powell 1974; Kornisch *et al.* 2019; Slorach and Noehr 1973). While it has been suggested that handedness and sex might influence the association between stuttering and dichotic listening performance (Foundas *et al.* 2004b), the general pattern of results suggests that this association is spurious at best. Meta-analytic integration of the published literature and new data collection in a larger sample is needed to resolve this question.

Functional hemispheric asymmetries in electrophysiological activity

So far, only few studies have used EEG to investigate hemispheric asymmetries in individuals who stutter. For example, EEG alpha asymmetries have been measured in individuals who stutter and non-stuttering controls before a reading task (Moore and Lang 1977). The authors reported a leftward asymmetry in controls, indicating the typical leftward asymmetry for language processing, whereas stutterers showed a lower alpha in the right hemisphere, indicating atypical rightward language lateralization. Three years later, a study by the same first author indicated similar results for EEG alpha asymmetries measured during presentation of speech, but also during presentation of connected non-linguistic stimuli (Moore and Haynes 1980). Subsequently, it was reported that male individuals who stutter showed a right-hemispheric alpha reduction/right-hemispheric activation asymmetry during presentation of words, while controls showed the typical leftward language dominance (Moore *et al.* 1982). Moreover, it was reported that non-stuttering controls show a leftward EEG alpha asymmetry in the posterior cortex, while no such asymmetry was observed in individuals who stutter (Wells and Moore 1990).

Taken together, the empirical evidence unequivocally suggests more right-hemispheric processing of language in individuals who stutter compared to non-stuttering controls. However, due to small sample sizes as well as the fact that most studies have been published decades ago, independent replication of these effects in larger cohorts is desirable.

Functional hemispheric asymmetries in brain activation

Hemispheric asymmetries in language processing in stuttering individuals have been assessed in a multitude of studies, beginning with early PET studies that showed that stuttering individuals did not show the typical leftward asymmetric activations associated with language (Braun *et al.* 1997; Fox *et al.* 1996). In 2005, a first ALE meta-analysis of imaging studies of chronic developmental stuttering in adults was published, integrating data from eight PET and fMRI studies, including those mentioned previously (Brown *et al.* 2005). Almost a decade later, the study by Brown *et al.* (2005) was updated in another ALE meta-analysis of 17 neuroimaging studies on speech processing in stutterers (Belyk *et al.* 2015). In this study, two different ALE meta-analyses were performed. First, the authors analysed trait stuttering by comparing activation maps of individuals who stutter to controls while speech was fluent. Second, the authors analysed state stuttering by comparing activation maps of individuals who stutter while they were stuttering compared to episodes of fluent speech from the same individuals. Trait stuttering was linked to a decreased likelihood of speech-related activation in the left larynx motor cortex and speech-relevant auditory areas in the temporal lobe. Moreover, trait stuttering was also linked to an increased likelihood of speech-related activation in several right-hemispheric areas. These included the right hemisphere homolog of Broca's area as well as several speech-relevant motor areas in the right hemisphere and several other frontal and parietal areas. Altogether, the meta-analytic data thus suggest a rightward shift during fluent speech production in individuals who stutter, compared to controls. Moreover, the analysis of trait stuttering suggested a more pronounced right-shift for stuttering compared to fluent speech in individuals who stutter. Overall, the most prominent activation decrease was observed in the left larynx motor cortex. Further left-hemispheric clusters that showed activation decreases were in several temporal lobe auditory areas and left cerebellar vermis.

Structural asymmetries in grey matter

A reduction of the typical leftward asymmetry of the PT, an important structure in the language network, has been reported for stuttering (Foundas *et al.* 2001). It has also shown that atypical asymmetries in stuttering are related to symptom severity, with individuals with an atypical rightward asymmetry of the PT showing more severe stuttering (Foundas *et al.* 2004a). In contrast, a more recent study in a larger sample of 67 individuals who stutter and 63 controls did not indicate any significant difference in PT asymmetry between the two groups (Gough *et al.* 2018). Moreover, another smaller study in 19 individuals who stutter and 16 controls reported that individuals who stutter showed typical patterns of cerebral asymmetry and that there were no significant differences between the two groups regarding frontal and occipital width asymmetry, frontal and occipital pole asymmetry, and

PT and Sylvian fissure asymmetries (Cykowski *et al.* 2008). These findings suggest that the effect of altered PT asymmetry in stuttering does not replicate well.

In addition to PT asymmetries, several other structural asymmetries in the grey matter have been reported in stuttering. One study, investigating 16 adults with persistent stuttering and 16 matched controls, found that control subjects showed a larger right than left prefrontal cortex and a larger left than right occipital lobe volume, while the stuttering individuals did not show these asymmetries (Foundas *et al.* 2003). Moreover, two studies that each compared 14 children who stuttered to controls reported that stuttering was associated with atypical asymmetries of brain torque (Mock *et al.* 2012) and an atypical leftward asymmetry of the caudate nucleus (Foundas *et al.* 2013).

Structural asymmetries in white matter

Surprisingly little research has been published on differences in structural white matter asymmetries between individuals who stutter and controls. One 2004 study compared white matter structure in ten adults who stuttered and ten controls (Jäncke *et al.* 2004). The authors reported a leftward white matter asymmetry in the auditory cortex that was absent in individuals who stutter. Moreover, individuals who stutter showed increased white matter volumes in a right-hemispheric network containing connections to several important structures in the language network, including the PT, pars triangularis, and the precentral gyrus close to the face and mouth representation. These findings provide preliminary evidence for altered hemispheric asymmetries in the white matter structures involved in the language network. However, the small cohort size of the study suggests that these results should only be interpreted cautiously and that independent replication in larger samples is needed.

Conclusion

Taken together, the empirical evidence suggests that stuttering is associated with altered functional hemispheric asymmetries in the language domain, while the motor domain remains unaffected. Both the EEG data and meta-analysis of functional imaging studies unequivocally suggest more rightward functional processing of language. Whether or not these functional changes are accompanied by changes in structural asymmetries in language-relevant grey matter areas is not clear. While several studies in small samples (typically less than 20 individuals who stutter) reported significant differences in language-relevant areas such as the PT, newer studies with null results question these findings. Certainly, more research in larger cohorts is needed in this area. The evidence on white matter structural asymmetries again suggests a rightward shift of language networks.

References

Alperin, B.R., *et al.*, 2019. The relationship between alpha asymmetry and ADHD depends on negative affect level and parenting practices. *Journal of Psychiatric Research*, 116, 138–146.

American Psychiatric Association, 2013. *Diagnostic and statistical manual of mental disorders. DSM-5.* 5th ed. Washington, DC: American Psychiatric Publishing.

Aoki, Y., *et al.*, 2013. Comparison of white matter integrity between autism spectrum disorder subjects and typically developing individuals: a meta-analysis of diffusion tensor imaging tractography studies. *Molecular Autism*, 4 (1), 25.

Arnett, A.B., *et al.*, 2017. Explaining the sex difference in dyslexia. *Journal of Child Psychology and Psychiatry, and Allied Disciplines*, 58 (6), 719–727.

Arning, L., *et al.*, 2013. PCSK6 VNTR polymorphism is associated with degree of handedness but not direction of handedness. *PLoS One*, 8 (6), e67251.

Asperger, H., 1944. Die Autistischen Psychopathen im Kindesalter. Trans. U. FRITH in U. FRITH (ed.). *Autism and Asperger Syndrome.* Cambridge: Cambridge University Press, 1991: 37–92. *Archiv für Psychiatrie und Nervenkrankheiten*, 117, 76–136.

Baker, K.F., Montgomery, A.A., and Abramson, R., 2010. Brief report: perception and lateralization of spoken emotion by youths with high-functioning forms of autism. *Journal of Autism and Developmental Disorders*, 40 (1), 123–129.

Banfi, C., *et al.*, 2019. White matter alterations and tract lateralization in children with dyslexia and isolated spelling deficits. *Human Brain Mapping*, 40 (3), 765–776.

Baving, L., Laucht, M., and Schmidt, M.H., 1999. Atypical frontal brain activation in ADHD: preschool and elementary school boys and girls. *Journal of the American Academy of Child and Adolescent Psychiatry*, 38 (11), 1363–1371.

Beaton, A.A., 1997. The relation of planum temporale asymmetry and morphology of the corpus callosum to handedness, gender, and dyslexia: a review of the evidence. *Brain and Language*, 60 (2), 255–322.

Belyk, M., Kraft, S.J., and Brown, S., 2015. Stuttering as a trait or state—an ALE meta-analysis of neuroimaging studies. *The European Journal of Neuroscience*, 41 (2), 275–284.

Berenbaum, S.A., and Denburg, S.D., 1995. Evaluating the empirical support for the role of testosterone in the Geschwind-Behan-Galaburda model of cerebral lateralization: commentary on Bryden, McManus, and Bulman-Fleming. *Brain and Cognition*, 27 (1), 79–83; discussion 94–97.

Bishop, D.V.M., 1990. *Handedness and developmental disorder*. Oxford and Philadelphia, PA: Mac Keith Press and J.B. Lippincott.

Bishop, D.V.M., 2013. Cerebral asymmetry and language development: cause, correlate, or consequence? *Science (New York, N.Y.)*, 340 (6138), 1230531.

Blackstock, E.G., 1978. Cerebral asymmetry and the development of early infantile autism. *Journal of Autism and Childhood Schizophrenia*, 8 (3), 339–353.

Bowers, D., and Heilman, K.M., 1980. Pseudoneglect: effects of hemispace on a tactile line bisection task. *Neuropsychologia*, 18 (4–5), 491–498.

Brandler, W.M., and Paracchini, S., 2014. The genetic relationship between handedness and neurodevelopmental disorders. *Trends in Molecular Medicine*, 20 (2), 83–90.

Braun, A.R., *et al.*, 1997. Altered patterns of cerebral activity during speech and language production in developmental stuttering. An $H_2(15)O$ positron emission tomography study. *Brain: A Journal of Neurology*, 120 (Pt 5), 761–784.

Brown, S., *et al.*, 2005. Stuttered and fluent speech production: an ALE meta-analysis of functional neuroimaging studies. *Human Brain Mapping*, 25 (1), 105–117.

Bryden, M.P., McManus, I.C., and Bulman-Fleming, M.B., 1994. Evaluating the empirical support for the Geschwind-Behan-Galaburda model of cerebral lateralization. *Brain and Cognition*, 26 (2), 103–167.

Burt, S.A., 2009. Rethinking environmental contributions to child and adolescent psychopathology: a meta-analysis of shared environmental influences. *Psychological Bulletin*, 135, 608–637.

Cardinale, R.C., *et al.*, 2013. Pervasive rightward asymmetry shifts of functional networks in autism spectrum disorder. *JAMA Psychiatry*, 70 (9), 975–982.

Carper, R.A., *et al.*, 2016. Reduced hemispheric asymmetry of White matter microstructure in autism spectrum disorder. *Journal of the American Academy of Child and Adolescent Psychiatry*, 55 (12), 1073–1080.

Carrion-Castillo, A., *et al.*, 2020. Genetic effects on planum temporale asymmetry and their limited relevance to neurodevelopmental disorders, intelligence or educational attainment. *Cortex; A Journal Devoted to the Study of the Nervous System and Behavior*, 124, 137–153.

Castellanos, F.X., *et al.*, 1994. Quantitative morphology of the caudate nucleus in attention deficit hyperactivity disorder. *The American Journal of Psychiatry*, 151 (12), 1791–1796.

Castellanos, F.X., *et al.*, 1996. Quantitative brain magnetic resonance imaging in attention-deficit hyperactivity disorder. *Archives of General Psychiatry*, 53 (7), 607–616.

Chandrasekar, G., *et al.*, 2013. The zebrafish orthologue of the dyslexia candidate gene DYX1C1 is essential for cilia growth and function. *PLoS One*, 8 (5), e63123.

Chaste, P., and Leboyer, M., 2012. Autism risk factors: genes, environment, and gene-environment interactions. *Dialogues in Clinical Neuroscience*, 14 (3), 281–292.

Chen, H., *et al.*, 2014. Stuttering candidate genes DRD2 but not SLC6A3 is associated with developmental dyslexia in Chinese population. *Behavioral and Brain Functions*, 10 (1), 29.

Chen, Q., *et al.*, 2017. Familial aggregation of attention-deficit/hyperactivity disorder. *Journal of Child Psychology and Psychiatry*, 58 (3), 231–239.

Chrysanthis, K., 1947. Stammering and handedness. *The Lancet*, 249 (6442), 270–271.

Conti, E., *et al.*, 2016. Lateralization of brain networks and clinical severity in toddlers with autism spectrum disorder: a HARDI diffusion MRI study. *Autism Research: Official Journal of the International Society for Autism Research*, 9 (3), 382–392.

Curry, F.K.W., and Gregory, H.H., 1969. The performance of stutterers on dichotic listening tasks thought to reflect cerebral dominance. *Journal of Speech and Hearing Research*, 12 (1), 73–82.

Cykowski, M.D., *et al.*, 2008. Perisylvian sulcal morphology and cerebral asymmetry patterns in adults who stutter. *Cerebral Cortex (New York, N.Y.: 1991)*, 18 (3), 571–583.

Dang, L.C., *et al.*, 2016. Caudate asymmetry is related to attentional impulsivity and an objective measure of ADHD-like attentional problems in healthy adults. *Brain Structure & Function*, 221 (1), 277–286.

Davidson, E.M., and Prior, M.R., 1978. Laterality and selective attention in hyperactive children. *Journal of Abnormal Child Psychology*, 6 (4), 475–481.

Demontis, D., *et al.*, 2019. Discovery of the first genome-wide significant risk loci for attention deficit/hyperactivity disorder. *Nature Genetics*, 51 (1), 63–75.

Dickstein, S.G., *et al.*, 2006. The neural correlates of attention deficit hyperactivity disorder: an ALE meta-analysis. *Journal of Child Psychology and Psychiatry*, 47 (10), 1051–1062.

Dorman, M.F., and Porter, R.J., 1975. Hemispheric lateralization for speech perception in stutterers. *Cortex*, 11 (2), 181–185.

Dougherty, C.C., *et al.*, 2016. Asymmetry of fusiform structure in autism spectrum disorder: trajectory and association with symptom severity. *Molecular Autism*, 7, 28.

Douglas, P.K., *et al.*, 2018. Hemispheric brain asymmetry differences in youths with attention-deficit/hyperactivity disorder. *NeuroImage. Clinical*, 18, 744–752.

Dramsdahl, M., *et al.*, 2011. Cognitive control in adults with attention-deficit/hyperactivity disorder. *Psychiatry Research*, 188 (3), 406–410.

Eckert, M.A., *et al.*, 2016. Gray matter features of reading disability: a combined meta-analytic and direct analysis approach(1,2,3,4). *eNeuro*, 3 (1).

Eglinton, E., and Annett, M., 1994. Handedness and dyslexia: a meta-analysis. *Perceptual and Motor Skills*, 79 (3 Pt 2), 1611–1616.

Ellison-Wright, I., Ellison-Wright, Z., and Bullmore, E., 2008. Structural brain change in attention deficit hyperactivity disorder identified by meta-analysis. *BMC Psychiatry*, 8, 51.

English, M.C.W., Maybery, M.T., and Visser, T.A.W., 2017. Reduced pseudon-eglect for physical space, but not mental representations of space, for adults with autistic traits. *Journal of Autism and Developmental Disorders*, 47 (7), 1956–1965.

Fabiano, G.A., *et al.*, 2009. A meta-analysis of behavioral treatments for attention-deficit/hyperactivity disorder. *Clinical Psychology Review*, 29 (2), 129–140.

Floris, D.L., *et al.*, 2016. Atypically rightward cerebral asymmetry in male adults with autism stratifies individuals with and without language delay. *Human Brain Mapping*, 37 (1), 230–253.

Foster, L.M., *et al.*, 2002. Planum temporale asymmetry and ear advantage in dichotic listening in developmental dyslexia and attention-deficit/hyperactivity disorder (ADHD). *Journal of the International Neuropsychological Society: JINS*, 8 (1), 22–36.

Foundas, A.L., *et al.*, 2001. Anomalous anatomy of speech-language areas in adults with persistent developmental stuttering. *Neurology*, 57 (2), 207–215.

Foundas, A.L., *et al.*, 2003. Atypical cerebral laterality in adults with persistent developmental stuttering. *Neurology*, 61 (10), 1378–1385.

Foundas, A.L., *et al.*, 2004a. Aberrant auditory processing and atypical planum temporale in developmental stuttering. *Neurology*, 63 (9), 1640–1646.

Foundas, A.L., *et al.*, 2004b. Verbal dichotic listening in developmental stuttering: subgroups with atypical auditory processing. *Cognitive and Behavioral Neurology: Official Journal of the Society for Behavioral and Cognitive Neurology*, 17 (4), 224–232.

Foundas, A.L., *et al.*, 2013. Atypical caudate anatomy in children who stutter. *Perceptual and Motor Skills*, 116 (2), 528–543.

Fox, P.T., *et al.*, 1996. A PET study of the neural systems of stuttering. *Nature*, 382 (6587), 158–161.

Froehlich, T.E., *et al.*, 2011. Update on environmental risk factors for attention-deficit/hyperactivity disorder. *Current Psychiatry Reports*, 13 (5), 333.

Fu, L., *et al.*, 2020. Longitudinal study of brain asymmetries in autism and developmental delays aged 2–5 years. *Neuroscience*, 432, 137–149.

Gabard-Durnam, L., *et al.*, 2015. Alpha asymmetry in infants at risk for autism spectrum disorders. *Journal of Autism and Developmental Disorders*, 45 (2), 473–480.

Galin, D., *et al.*, 1988. EEG alpha asymmetry in dyslexics during speaking and block design tasks. *Brain and Language*, 35 (2), 241–253.

Geschwind, N., and Behan, P., 1982. Left-handedness: association with immune disease, migraine, and developmental learning disorder. *Proceedings of the National Academy of Sciences of the United States of America*, 79 (16), 5097–5100.

Geschwind, N., and Galaburda, A.M., 1985a. Cerebral lateralization. Biological mechanisms, associations, and pathology: I. A hypothesis and a program for research. *Archives of Neurology*, 42 (5), 428–459.

Geschwind, N., and Galaburda, A.M., 1985b. Cerebral lateralization. Biological mechanisms, associations, and pathology: II. A hypothesis and a program for research. *Archives of Neurology*, 42 (6), 521–552.

Geschwind, N., and Galaburda, A.M., 1985c. Cerebral lateralization. Biological mechanisms, associations, and pathology: III. A hypothesis and a program for research. *Archives of Neurology*, 42 (7), 634–654.

Gold, R., and Faust, M., 2010. Right hemisphere dysfunction and metaphor comprehension in young adults with Asperger syndrome. *Journal of Autism and Developmental Disorders*, 40 (7), 800–811.

Gough, P.M., *et al.*, 2018. Planum temporale asymmetry in people who stutter. *Journal of Fluency Disorders*, 55, 94–105.

Grabrucker, S., *et al.*, 2017. Brain lateralization in mice is associated with Zinc signaling and altered in prenatal Zinc deficient mice that display features of autism spectrum disorder. *Frontiers in Molecular Neuroscience*, 10, 450.

Gruber, L., and Powell, R.L., 1974. Responses of stuttering and non-stuttering children to a dichotic listening task. *Perceptual and Motor Skills*, 38 (1), 263–264.

De Guibert, C., *et al.*, 2011. Abnormal functional lateralization and activity of language brain areas in typical specific language impairment (developmental dysphasia). *Brain: A Journal of Neurology*, 134 (Pt 10), 3044–3058.

Hakvoort, B., *et al.*, 2016. Dichotic listening as an index of lateralization of speech perception in familial risk children with and without dyslexia. *Brain and Cognition*, 109, 75–83.

Hale, T.S., *et al.*, 2006. Atypical brain laterality in adults with ADHD during dichotic listening for emotional intonation and words. *Neuropsychologia*, 44 (6), 896–904.

Hale, T.S., *et al.*, 2009a. Atypical alpha asymmetry in adults with ADHD. *Neuropsychologia*, 47 (10), 2082–2088.

Hale, T.S., *et al.*, 2009b. Rethinking a right hemisphere deficit in ADHD. *Journal of Attention Disorders*, 13 (1), 3–17.

Hale, T.S., *et al.*, 2010. Atypical EEG beta asymmetry in adults with ADHD. *Neuropsychologia*, 48 (12), 3532–3539.

Hale, T.S., *et al.*, 2014. Abnormal parietal brain function in ADHD: replication and extension of previous EEG beta asymmetry findings. *Frontiers in Psychiatry*, 5, 87.

Hasler, R., *et al.*, 2017. Inter-hemispherical asymmetry in default-mode functional connectivity and BAIAP2 gene are associated with anger expression in ADHD adults. *Psychiatry Research. Neuroimaging*, 269, 54–61.

Hayashi, M., *et al.*, 1989. A neurolinguistic study of autistic children employing dichotic listening. *The Tokai Journal of Experimental and Clinical Medicine*, 14 (4), 339–345.

Heiervang, E., *et al.*, 2000. Planum temporale, planum parietale and dichotic listening in dyslexia. *Neuropsychologia*, 38 (13), 1704–1713.

Heilman, K.M., *et al.*, 1986. The right hemisphere: neuropsychological functions. *Journal of Neurosurgery*, 64 (5), 693–704.

Heilman, K.M., and van den Abell, T., 1980. Right hemisphere dominance for attention: the mechanism underlying hemispheric asymmetries of inattention (neglect). *Neurology*, 30 (3), 327–330.

Heilman, K.M., Voeller, K.K., and Nadeau, S.E., 1991. A possible pathophysiologic substrate of attention deficit hyperactivity disorder. *Journal of Child Neurology*, 6 (Suppl.), S76–S81.

Helfer, B., *et al.*, 2020. Lateralization of attention in adults with ADHD: evidence of pseudoneglect. *European Psychiatry: The Journal of the Association of European Psychiatrists*, 63 (1), e68.

Helland, T., *et al.*, 2008. Dichotic listening and school performance in dyslexia. *Dyslexia (Chichester, England)*, 14 (1), 42–53.

Herringshaw, A.J., *et al.*, 2016. Hemispheric differences in language processing in autism spectrum disorders: a meta-analysis of neuroimaging studies. *Autism Research: Official Journal of the International Society for Autism Research*, 9 (10), 1046–1057.

Hohagen, F., and Voderholzer, U., eds., 2019. *Therapie psychischer Erkrankungen [Therapy of mental illnesses]. State of the art.* 14th ed. München, Deutschland: Elsevier.

Hugdahl, K., *et al.*, 1995. Absence of ear advantage on the consonant-vowel dichotic listening test in adolescent and adult dyslexics: specific auditory-phonetic dysfunction. *Journal of Clinical and Experimental Neuropsychology*, 17 (6), 833–840.

Jäncke, L., Hänggi, J., and Steinmetz, H., 2004. Morphological brain differences between adult stutterers and non-stutterers. *BMC Neurology*, 4 (1), 23.

Jewell, G., and McCourt, M.E., 2000. Pseudoneglect: a review and meta-analysis of performance factors in line bisection tasks. *Neuropsychologia*, 38 (1), 93–110.

Joseph, R.M., *et al.*, 2014. Structural asymmetries of language-related gray and white matter and their relationship to language function in young children with ASD. *Brain Imaging and Behavior*, 8 (1), 60–72.

Jouravlev, O., *et al.*, 2020. Reduced language lateralization in autism and the broader autism phenotype as assessed with robust individual-subjects analyses. *Autism Research: Official Journal of the International Society for Autism Research*, 13, 1746–1761.

Kanner, L., 1943. Autistic disturbances of affective contact. *Nervous Child*, 2 (3), 217–250.

Klimkeit, E.I., *et al.*, 2003. Perceptual asymmetries in normal children and children with attention deficit/hyperactivity disorder. *Brain and Cognition*, 52 (2), 205–215.

Klimkeit, E.I., and Bradshaw, J.L., 2006. Anomalous lateralisation in neurodevelopmental disorders. *Cortex*, 42 (1), 113–116.

Knaus, T.A., *et al.*, 2012. Prefrontal and occipital asymmetry and volume in boys with autism spectrum disorder. *Cognitive and Behavioral Neurology: Official Journal of the Society for Behavioral and Cognitive Neurology*, 25 (4), 186–194.

Kornisch, M., Robb, M.P., and Jones, R.D., 2020. Estimates of functional cerebral hemispheric differences in monolingual and bilingual people who stutter: dichotic listening paradigm. *Clinical Linguistics & Phonetics*, 34, 774–789.

Kraft, S.J., and Yairi, E., 2012. Genetic bases of stuttering: the state of the art, 2011. *Folia phoniatrica et logopaedica: Official Organ of the International Association of Logopedics and Phoniatrics (IALP)*, 64 (1), 34–47.

Kushner, H.I., 2012. Retraining left-handers and the aetiology of stuttering: the rise and fall of an intriguing theory. *Laterality*, 17 (6), 673–693.

Lange, N., *et al.*, 2010. Atypical diffusion tensor hemispheric asymmetry in autism. *Autism Research: Official Journal of the International Society for Autism Research*, 3 (6), 350–358.

Li, D., *et al.*, 2019. Reduced hemispheric asymmetry of brain anatomical networks in attention deficit hyperactivity disorder. *Brain Imaging and Behavior*, 13 (3), 669–684.

Lin, H.-L., and Tsuang, H.-C., 2018. Handedness and attention deficit/hyperactivity disorder symptoms in college students. *The Psychiatric Quarterly*, 89 (1), 103–110.

Lindell, A.K., and Hudry, K., 2013. Atypicalities in cortical structure, handedness, and functional lateralization for language in autism spectrum disorders. *Neuropsychology Review*, 23 (3), 257–270.

Linkersdörfer, J., *et al.*, 2012. Grey matter alterations co-localize with functional abnormalities in developmental dyslexia: an ALE meta-analysis. *PLoS One*, 7 (8), e43122.

Maisog, J.M., *et al.*, 2008. A meta-analysis of functional neuroimaging studies of dyslexia. *Annals of the New York Academy of Sciences*, 1145, 237–259.

Markou, P., Ahtam, B., and Papadatou-Pastou, M., 2017. Elevated levels of atypical handedness in autism: meta-analyses. *Neuropsychology Review*, 27 (3), 258–283.

Martínez, J.A., and Sánchez, E., 1999. Dichotic listening CV lateralization and developmental dyslexia. *Journal of Clinical and Experimental Neuropsychology*, 21 (4), 519–534.

Masi, A., *et al.*, 2017. An overview of autism spectrum disorder, heterogeneity and treatment options. *Neuroscience Bulletin*, 33 (2), 183–193.

Massinen, S., *et al.*, 2011. Increased expression of the dyslexia candidate gene DCDC2 affects length and signaling of primary cilia in neurons. *PLoS One*, 6 (6), e20580.

McKeever, W.F., and VanDeventer, A.D., 1975. Dyslexic adolescents: evidence of impaired visual and auditory language processing associated with normal lateralization and visual responsivity. *Cortex*, 11 (4), 361–378.

Mock, J.R., *et al.*, 2012. Atypical brain torque in boys with developmental stuttering. *Developmental Neuropsychology*, 37 (5), 434–452.

Moore, W.H., Craven, D.C., and Faber, M.M., 1982. Hemispheric alpha asymmetries of words with positive, negative, and neutral arousal values preceding tasks of recall and recognition: electrophysiological and behavioral results from stuttering males and nonstuttering males and females. *Brain and Language*, 17 (2), 211–224.

Moore, W.H., and Haynes, W.O., 1980. Alpha hemispheric asymmetry and stuttering: some support for a segmentation dysfunction hypothesis. *Journal of Speech and Hearing Research*, 23 (2), 229–247.

Moore, W.H., and Lang, M.K., 1977. Alpha asymmetry over the right and left hemispheres of stutterers and control subjects preceding massed oral readings: a preliminary investigation. *Perceptual and Motor Skills*, 44 (1), 223–230.

Nastou, E., Ocklenburg, S., and Papadatou-Pastou, M., 2020. *Handedness in ADHD: meta-analyses*. PsyArXiv. July 15. doi: 10.31234/osf.io/zyrvg.

Neumann, K., *et al.*, 2017. The pathogenesis, assessment and treatment of speech fluency disorders. *Deutsches Arzteblatt International*, 114 (22–23), 383–390.

Obrzut, J.E., and Boliek, C.A., 1986. Lateralization characteristics in learning disabled children. *Journal of Learning Disabilities*, 19 (5), 308–314.

Ogawa, T., *et al.*, 1982. Ontogenic development of EEG-asymmetry in early infantile autism. *Brain & Development*, 4 (6), 439–449.

Orton, S.T., 1937. *Reading, writing and speech problems in children*. New York, NY: W. W. Norton & Company.

Paclt, I., *et al.*, 2016. Reverse asymmetry and changes in brain structural volume of the basal ganglia in ADHD, developmental changes and the impact of stimulant medications. *Neuro Endocrinology Letters*, 37 (1), 29–32.

Papadatou-Pastou, M., *et al.*, 2020. Human handedness: a meta-analysis. *Psychological Bulletin*, 146 (6), 481–524.

Papagiannopoulou, E.A., and Lagopoulos, J., 2016. Resting state EEG hemispheric power asymmetry in children with dyslexia. *Frontiers in Pediatrics*, 4, 11.

Patterson, P.H., 2011. Maternal infection and immune involvement in autism. *Trends in Molecular Medicine*, 17 (7), 389–394.

Paulesu, E., Danelli, L., and Berlingeri, M., 2014. Reading the dyslexic brain: multiple dysfunctional routes revealed by a new meta-analysis of PET and fMRI activation studies. *Frontiers in Human Neuroscience*, 8, 830.

Penolazzi, B., Spironelli, C., and Angrilli, A., 2008. Delta EEG activity as a marker of dysfunctional linguistic processing in developmental dyslexia. *Psychophysiology*, 45 (6), 1025–1033.

Peters, M., Reimers, S., and Manning, J.T., 2006. Hand preference for writing and associations with selected demographic and behavioral variables in 255,100 subjects: the BBC internet study. *Brain and Cognition*, 62 (2), 177–189.

Pollack, C., Luk, G., and Christodoulou, J.A., 2015. A meta-analysis of functional reading systems in typically developing and struggling readers across different alphabetic languages. *Frontiers in Psychology*, 6, 191.

Postema, M.C., *et al.*, 2019. Altered structural brain asymmetry in autism spectrum disorder in a study of 54 datasets. *Nature Communications*, 10 (1), 4958.

Preslar, J., *et al.*, 2014. Autism, lateralisation, and handedness: a review of the literature and meta-analysis. *Laterality*, 19 (1), 64–95.

Previc, F.H., 1994. Assessing the legacy of the GBG model. *Brain and Cognition*, 26 (2), 174–180.

Prior, M.R., and Bradshaw, J.L., 1979. Hemisphere functioning in autistic children. *Cortex*, 15 (1), 73–81.

Ramtekkar, U.P., *et al.*, 2010. Sex and age differences in attention-deficit/hyperactivity disorder symptoms and diagnoses: implications for DSM-V and ICD-11.

Journal of the American Academy of Child and Adolescent Psychiatry, 49 (3), 217–228.e1–3.

Ribasés, M., *et al.*, 2009. Case-control study of six genes asymmetrically expressed in the two cerebral hemispheres: association of BAIAP2 with attention-deficit/ hyperactivity disorder. *Biological Psychiatry*, 66 (10), 926–934.

Richlan, F., Kronbichler, M., and Wimmer, H., 2009. Functional abnormalities in the dyslexic brain: a quantitative meta-analysis of neuroimaging studies. *Human Brain Mapping*, 30 (10), 3299–3308.

Robinson, K.J., *et al.*, 2016. The PCSK6 gene is associated with handedness, the autism spectrum, and magical ideation in a non-clinical population. *Neuropsychologia*, 84, 205–212.

Rolfe, M.H.S., Hausmann, M., and Waldie, K.E., 2006. Hemispheric functioning in children with subtypes of attention-deficit/hyperactivity disorder. *Journal of Attention Disorders*, 10 (1), 20–27.

Rysstad, A.L., and Pedersen, A.V., 2016. Brief report: non-right-handedness within the autism spectrum disorder. *Journal of Autism and Developmental Disorders*, 46 (3), 1110–1117.

Samea, F., *et al.*, 2019. Brain alterations in children/adolescents with ADHD revisited: a neuroimaging meta-analysis of 96 structural and functional studies. *Neuroscience and Biobehavioral Reviews*, 100, 1–8.

Scerri, T.S., *et al.*, 2011. PCSK6 is associated with handedness in individuals with dyslexia. *Human Molecular Genetics*, 20 (3), 608–614.

Schmitz, J., *et al.*, 2018. KIAA0319 promoter DNA methylation predicts dichotic listening performance in forced-attention conditions. *Behavioural Brain Research*, 337, 1–7.

Schrimsher, G.W., *et al.*, 2002. Caudate nucleus volume asymmetry predicts attention-deficit hyperactivity disorder (ADHD) symptomatology in children. *Journal of Child Neurology*, 17 (12), 877–884.

Schulte-Körne, G., 2010. The prevention, diagnosis, and treatment of dyslexia. *Deutsches Arzteblatt International*, 107 (41), 718–726; quiz 27.

Segal, D., Shalev, L., and Mashal, N., 2017. Attenuated hemispheric asymmetry in metaphor processing among adults with ADHD. *Neuropsychology*, 31 (6), 636–647.

Shapleske, J., *et al.*, 1999. The planum temporale: a systematic, quantitative review of its structural, functional and clinical significance. *Brain Research. Brain Research Reviews*, 29 (1), 26–49.

Shaw, P., *et al.*, 2009. Development of cortical asymmetry in typically developing children and its disruption in attention-deficit/hyperactivity disorder. *Archives of General Psychiatry*, 66 (8), 888–896.

Sheppard, D.M., *et al.*, 1999. Effects of stimulant medication on the lateralisation of line bisection judgements of children with attention deficit hyperactivity disorder. *Journal of Neurology, Neurosurgery, and Psychiatry*, 66 (1), 57–63.

Silk, T.J., *et al.*, 2016. Abnormal asymmetry in frontostriatal white matter in children with attention deficit hyperactivity disorder. *Brain Imaging and Behavior*, 10 (4), 1080–1089.

Slorach, N., and Noehr, B., 1973. Dichotic listening in stuttering and dyslalic children. *Cortex*, 9 (3), 295–300.

Sommers, R.K., Brady, W.A., and Moore, W.H., 1975. Dichotic ear preferences of stuttering children and adults. *Perceptual and Motor Skills*, 41 (3), 931–938.

Spironelli, C., et al., 2006. Inverted EEG theta lateralization in dyslexic children during phonological processing. *Neuropsychologia*, 44 (14), 2814–2821.

Spironelli, C., Penolazzi, B., and Angrilli, A., 2008. Dysfunctional hemispheric asymmetry of theta and beta EEG activity during linguistic tasks in developmental dyslexia. *Biological Psychology*, 77 (2), 123–131.

Stefanatos, G.A., and Wasserstein, J., 2001. Attention deficit/hyperactivity disorder as a right hemisphere syndrome. Selective literature review and detailed neuropsychological case studies. *Annals of the New York Academy of Sciences*, 931, 172–195.

Strub, R.L., Black, F.W., and Naeser, M.A., 1987. Anomalous dominance in sibling stutterers: evidence from CT scan asymmetries, dichotic listening, neuropsychological testing, and handedness. *Brain and Language*, 30 (2), 338–350.

Sun, Y.-F., Lee, J.-S., and Kirby, R., 2010. Brain imaging findings in dyslexia. *Pediatrics and Neonatology*, 51 (2), 89–96.

Uhlíkova, P., et al., 2007. Asymmetry of basal ganglia in children with attention deficit hyperactivity disorder. *Neuro Endocrinology Letters*, 28 (5), 604–609.

Vandermosten, M., et al., 2012. A qualitative and quantitative review of diffusion tensor imaging studies in reading and dyslexia. *Neuroscience and Biobehavioral Reviews*, 36 (6), 1532–1552.

Vandermosten, M., et al., 2013. White matter lateralization and interhemispheric coherence to auditory modulations in normal reading and dyslexic adults. *Neuropsychologia*, 51 (11), 2087–2099.

van Strien, J.W., Bouma, A., and Bakker, D.J., 1987. Birth stress, autoimmune diseases, and handedness. *Journal of Clinical and Experimental Neuropsychology*, 9 (6), 775–780.

Wan, C.Y., et al., 2012. Atypical hemispheric asymmetry in the arcuate fasciculus of completely nonverbal children with autism. *Annals of the New York Academy of Sciences*, 1252, 332–337.

Webster, W.G., and Poulos, M., 1987. Handedness distributions among adults who stutter. *Cortex*, 23 (4), 705–708.

Weikard, M.A., 1775–77. *Der philosophische Arzt [The philosophical doctor]*. Frankfurt & Berlin: in der Andreaischen Buchhandlung.

Wells, B.G., and Moore, W.H., 1990. EEG alpha asymmetries in stutterers and non-stutterers: effects of linguistic variables on hemispheric processing and fluency. *Neuropsychologia*, 28 (12), 1295–1305.

Werling, D.M., and Geschwind, D.H., 2013. Sex differences in autism spectrum disorders. *Current Opinion in Neurology*, 26 (2), 146–153.

WHO, 2016. International classification of disease-10.

Wigal, S.B., 2009. Efficacy and safety limitations of attention-deficit hyperactivity disorder pharmacotherapy in children and adults. *CNS Drugs*, 23 (Suppl. 1), 21–31.

Wu, Z.-M., *et al.*, 2020. Altered brain white matter microstructural asymmetry in children with ADHD. *Psychiatry Research*, 285, 112817.

Zhao, J., *et al.*, 2016. Altered hemispheric lateralization of white matter pathways in developmental dyslexia: evidence from spherical deconvolution tractography. *Cortex; A Journal Devoted to the Study of the Nervous System and Behavior*, 76, 51–62.

3 Lateralization in psychiatric disorders

Introduction

Psychiatric disorders are typically defined by a normal early development with symptom onset mostly in adolescence and the first diagnosis in late adolescence to early adulthood. For the mentioned disorders besides substance-related and addictive disorders, onset in childhood is possible. As the symptom onset frequently co-occurs with behavioural changes occurring in adolescence, the first episode of the disorder is frequently diagnosed retrospectively. A genetic predisposition is believed to exist in many cases, but usually, an environmental factor, a so-called "second hit", leads to the onset of symptoms.

Schizophrenia

Definition of the disorder

The most widely studied psychiatric disorder in laterality research is schizophrenia. Roughly translated to "splitting of the mind", schizophrenia was named and characterized by Eugen Bleuler, a Swiss psychiatrist, in 1908 (Bleuler 1908). He intended to describe the dysfunction between personality, thinking, memory, and perception experienced by patients as an independent syndrome, which he called schizophrenia.

The symptoms of schizophrenia are categorized into positive and negative symptoms. Positive symptoms are hallucinations, motor problems, delusions of thought, and speech disorders whereas negative symptoms are characterized by flat affect, odd behaviour, apathy, self-neglect, anxiety, and/or social withdrawal (Elert 2014). Two of the criteria have to be present over at least one month for being diagnosed with schizophrenia (American Psychiatric Association 2013).

Around 0.3–0.7% of the global population is affected by schizophrenia at some point in their life (van Os and Kapur 2009). Schizophrenia occurs 1.4

times more frequently in males than in females and has an earlier onset in men (Picchioni and Murray 2007). Peak ages of onset are 25 years for males and 27 years for females (Cascio *et al.* 2012). Three-quarters of people diagnosed with schizophrenia suffer a recurrent relapse and ongoing disability. Symptom severity also depends on social background and whether or not the first treatment was delayed (Barry *et al.* 2012).

Genetic factors (Schizophrenia Working Group of the Psychiatric Genomics Consortium 2014; Pardiñas *et al.* 2018), as well as environmental factors, such as disruptions during neuronal growth or maternal infection during the second trimester of pregnancy, increase the risk to develop schizophrenia (Insel 2010). Cannabis, for example, is known to increase the risk for people who already carry other predisposing factors (Parakh and Basu 2013). Other substances, such as cocaine or amphetamines, can cause a psychosis-like state similar to that experienced in schizophrenia but do not seem to increase the risk (Picchioni and Murray 2007).

For the primary treatment of schizophrenia, antipsychotics are recommended which are especially efficient against positive symptoms (Remington *et al.* 2017). Psychological interventions, such as cognitive behavioural therapy, might be helpful for treatment adherence and psychoeducation for handling the symptoms, but medication is the first treatment option (Health Quality Ontario 2018).

So far, researchers, clinicians, and psychologists have been trying to understand the neuronal correlates of schizophrenia, especially disruptions that might lead to psychotic experiences such as hearing voices or the feeling of being controlled by someone else. Since the nineteenth century, the idea that disruptions in brain asymmetry could cause schizophrenia symptoms has been discussed in psychiatric research (Wigan 1844). In 1969, the psychiatrist Pierre Flor-Henry investigated a link between psychosis and temporal lobe epilepsy. When comparing the laterality of epileptic foci in epilepsy patients with and without schizophrenia, he found an overrepresentation of left-sided foci (right hemisphere: 9.5%; left hemisphere 43%; bilateral 47.5%) in epilepsy patients with schizophrenia compared to non-psychotic epilepsy patients (right hemisphere: 44%; left hemisphere: 22%; bilateral: 33%). Thus, disturbances of the language-dominant left hemisphere seemed to be related to schizophrenia, whereas the distribution of foci was random in non-psychotic patients (Flor-Henry 1969). This highly interesting finding gave rise to a steadily increasing number of laterality studies in patients with schizophrenia.

Handedness

One of the most replicated findings in clinical laterality research is the fact that non-right-handedness (e.g. left-handedness or mixed-handedness) is more common in patients with schizophrenia than in healthy controls. This was confirmed by several meta-analyses (Moher *et al.* 2009).

The first of these meta-analyses was conducted by Sommer and colleagues (Sommer *et al.* 2001a) who integrated 19 studies on handedness in schizophrenia. They found that non-right-handedness was more common in patients with schizophrenia than in healthy controls (odds ratio: 1.61) but also compared to psychiatric controls with other disorders than schizophrenia (odds ratio: 1.54). A few years later, a larger meta-analysis integrating 40 studies found that patients with schizophrenia had a significantly higher prevalence of left-handedness (odds ratio: 1.85), mixed-handedness (odds ratio: 1.77), and non-right-handedness (odds ratio: 1.58) compared to healthy controls (Dragovic and Hammond 2005). In the most recent meta-analysis on handedness in schizophrenia, 50 studies were integrated (Hirnstein and Hugdahl 2014). Here, the authors specifically investigated whether the higher rate of non-right-handedness in schizophrenia could be a gender effect, as males are more likely to be left-handed than females (Papadatou-Pastou *et al.* 2008) and patients with schizophrenia are also more likely to be male than female (Eranti *et al.* 2013). However, the meta-analysis clearly showed that both male (odds ratio: 1.5) and female (odds ratio: 1.63) patients with schizophrenia have an elevated rate of non-right-handedness compared to healthy controls.

In addition to these findings in patients with schizophrenia, individuals with high schizotypy also have a higher incidence of non-right-handedness than the general population. Schizotypy is a personality organization that harbours a liability to develop schizophrenia (Lenzenweger 2018). A meta-analysis of 12 studies with a total of 10,058 subjects (Somers *et al.* 2009) showed that non-right-handed participants (excluding strong left-handers) had higher schizotypy scores than right-handers. Interestingly, it has been shown that the imprinted gene *LRRTM1* mediates both schizotypy and handedness (Leach *et al.* 2014), providing a potential molecular link for the association between this personality trait and handedness. Besides, it was shown that mixed-footedness is more common in individuals with high schizotypy scores (Tran *et al.* 2015).

Psychophysiological paradigms

Handedness is not the only form of altered functional hemispheric asymmetries in schizophrenia. There is also strong empirical evidence suggesting that atypical (e.g. non-leftward) language lateralization is more common in patients with schizophrenia than in the general population (Ocklenburg *et al.* 2015). The most commonly used behavioural paradigm to compare language lateralization in patients with schizophrenia to healthy controls has been the dichotic listening task (Hugdahl 2000; Tervaniemi and Hugdahl 2003; Westerhausen and Kompus 2018).

Sommer and colleagues (Sommer *et al.* 2001a) performed a meta-analysis of ten studies using the dichotic listening task in patients with schizophrenia. The meta-analysis did not find that patients with schizophrenia had a reduced right ear advantage (REA). However, a second analysis, in which only the two versions of the dichotic listening task that are thought to reflect language lateralization most accurately (the fused words and the consonant vowel dichotic listening task) were included, revealed that patients with schizophrenia showed a reduced REA.

This is also in line with the results of the second meta-analysis of dichotic listening performance in patients with schizophrenia that was published more than a decade later (Ocklenburg *et al.* 2013). Here, it was shown that patients with schizophrenia showed reduced language lateralization compared to healthy controls, but the effect size was small. Additionally, the authors performed another analysis in which they compared patients who experienced auditory verbal hallucinations to non-hallucinating controls. Here, the effect size was substantially larger, indicating that patients who experienced hallucinations showed a greater reduction of the REA than patients with schizophrenia in general. This demonstrates that not all patients with schizophrenia experience the same reduction of language lateralization. Instead, those that experience symptoms that specifically affect the language system encounter a greater reduction of language lateralization. This symptom-specific approach to the relation of schizophrenia and lateralization (Ocklenburg *et al.* 2015) is also supported by other dichotic listening studies. For example, it has been shown that patients with low symptom severity and no experience of auditory verbal hallucinations might not even show a reduction of the REA (Løberg *et al.* 2002).

The dichotic listening task is not the only psychophysiological paradigm that has shown altered language lateralization in patients with schizophrenia. One study using the divided visual field paradigm (Bourne 2006) found that in a visual word recognition task, healthy controls showed significantly higher accuracy for the right visual field/the left hemisphere than for the left visual field/the right hemisphere (Min and Oh 1992). In contrast, patients with schizophrenia showed similar performances with both hemispheres, indicating a reduction of typical leftward language lateralization in line with the dichotic listening data.

Functional hemispheric asymmetries in electrophysiological activity

In addition to behavioural measures, several neuroscientific techniques have been used to investigate altered functional hemispheric asymmetries in schizophrenia (Oertel-Knöchel and Linden 2011; Oertel-Knöchel *et al.* 2012). One of the core research fields regarding the relation of hemispheric asymmetries and psychiatric disorders is changes in electroencephalography (EEG) alpha band asymmetries (Coan and Allen 2004; Smith *et al.* 2017). Here, it was found that patients with schizophrenia show greater left-lateralized alpha power than a large cohort of healthy controls, suggesting a deficit in left frontal activity at rest in patients (Gordon *et al.* 2010). The authors suggested that this pattern of EEG alpha asymmetry might be related to disconnections across wider frontotemporal networks. Interestingly, some EEG studies also suggest a role of symptom severity for asymmetry reduction in schizophrenia. For example, it was shown that an attenuation of the rightward EEG alpha asymmetries in patients with schizophrenia increased with the duration of the disease and correlated with the severity of negative symptoms (Jalili *et al.* 2010). Similar relations have also been found for EEG gamma band asymmetries. Here, it was reported that in schizophrenia patients, left hypofrontality during phonological processing was positively correlated with the severity of positive schizophrenia symptoms, specifically delusions and hallucinations (Spironelli and Angrilli 2015). Thus, in line with the dichotic listening data, EEG data suggest that symptom severity is a critical factor when it comes to the extent of atypical asymmetries in schizophrenia patients.

Functional hemispheric asymmetries in brain activation

Altered hemispheric asymmetries in schizophrenia have also been investigated concerning variations in regional cerebral blood flow measured with positron emission tomography (PET). Here, it was found that compared to healthy controls, patients with schizophrenia showed lower activation in the left frontal cortex, atypical activations in the right inferior frontal lobe, and weaker right inferior parietal deactivation during word production (Artiges *et al.* 2000). This finding is in line with the dichotic listening findings indicating less leftward language lateralization in schizophrenia patients.

One of the main techniques that have been employed to investigate altered hemispheric asymmetries in schizophrenia is functional magnetic resonance imaging (fMRI). Both resting state and task-related fMRI studies have been conducted in patients with schizophrenia. For resting-state fMRI, a recent study in 180 patients with schizophrenia and 358 healthy controls showed increased leftward lateralization of functional connectivity in patients with schizophrenia compared to healthy controls in most brain regions (Xie *et al.* 2018). This resting-state asymmetry seems to be related to symptom severity. For example, it was shown that patients who exhibited predominantly positive symptoms showed an increased leftward asymmetry of functional connectivity (Ke *et al.* 2010). However, not all studies show a more leftward asymmetry of functional connectivity in patients with schizophrenia.

In contrast, it has also been reported that patients with schizophrenia show reduced and not increased leftward resting-state connectivity compared to healthy controls (Agcaoglu *et al.* 2018). Therefore, more research is needed before any final conclusions about asymmetries of functional connectivity in schizophrenia can be made.

For task-related fMRI, the first landmark studies on altered hemispheric asymmetries in schizophrenia have been conducted by the group of Iris Sommer (Sommer *et al.* 2001b, 2003) on language lateralization. These studies showed that in both male and female patients with schizophrenia, language processing is less lateralized due to stronger activations in the right hemisphere compared to healthy controls. The decrease in language lateralization was significantly correlated with hallucination severity. Based on the results, Sommer proposed that decreased language lateralization in schizophrenia is the result of a failure to inhibit the non-dominant right hemisphere (Sommer and Kahn 2009). Following up on these initial studies, several authors replicated the finding of reduced lateralization in schizophrenia for brain activations in both the inferior frontal and the temporal lobe during speech processing (Alary *et al.* 2013; Bleich-Cohen *et al.* 2012; Dollfus *et al.* 2005; Razafimandimby *et al.* 2007; Weiss *et al.* 2004, 2006).

Structural hemispheric asymmetries in grey matter

Given the large number of studies showing altered functional hemispheric asymmetries in schizophrenia, it comes as no surprise that several researchers investigated schizophrenia-related changes in structural asymmetries in grey matter areas of the human brain. One key finding is that compared to healthy controls, patients with schizophrenia show a reduced leftward asymmetry of the planum temporale (PT), a brain area located posterior to the auditory cortex that contains Wernicke's area (Sommer *et al.* 2001a; Shapleske *et al.* 1999). Interestingly, it has been shown that the amount of the decrease of leftward PT asymmetry correlates with symptom severity (Oertel *et al.* 2010).

Hemispheric asymmetries in white matter and structural connectivity

In addition to changes in structural asymmetries in grey matter areas, schizophrenia has also been linked to altered hemispheric asymmetries in specific white matter tracts and structural connectivity in general. It has been shown that patients with schizophrenia show attenuated asymmetries of both functional and structural connectivity (Ribolsi *et al.* 2014). Interestingly, reduced asymmetry in brain anatomical network topology has been associated with the duration of illness and also whether or not patients show psychotic psychopathology (Sun *et al.* 2017). This again supports the idea of a link between symptom severity and altered hemispheric asymmetries (Ocklenburg *et al.* 2015).

Laterality changes have also been reported for specific white matter tracts. For example, it has been shown that patients with schizophrenia exhibit reduced leftward lateralization of white matter integrity in the frontal arcuate fasciculus, but stronger leftward asymmetries in the temporal arcuate fasciculus (Abdul-Rahman *et al.* 2012). These changes in structural white matter laterality correlated with the severity of positive psychotic symptoms, such as delusions and hallucinations. This relation between changes in arcuate fasciculus laterality and positive symptoms was also supported by a meta-analysis that compared patients with schizophrenia who experienced auditory verbal hallucinations to healthy controls (Geoffroy *et al.* 2014). Here, it was found that hallucinators showed reduced white matter integrity of the left arcuate fasciculus compared to controls. Besides, altered asymmetries of white matter structure have also been reported for the uncinate fasciculus. Here, a lack of the typical leftward asymmetry of white matter integrity was found in patients diagnosed with schizophrenia (Kubicki *et al.* 2002).

Theoretical accounts for the links between altered hemispheric asymmetries and schizophrenia

Over the years, several theoretical accounts have been brought forward to explain the link between schizophrenia and altered hemispheric asymmetries. These accounts vary in the extent to which they propose that atypical hemispheric asymmetries are a cause, consequence, or biological correlate of schizophrenia. While some theories like the hemispheric imbalance theory (Gruzelier 1994; Gruzelier *et al.* 1999) or the "Big Bang theory of the origin of schizophrenia and its relation to altered language asymmetries" (Crow 2008) assume that schizophrenia can develop from a breakdown of typical asymmetrical brain organization, most researchers today do not assume that atypical asymmetries directly cause schizophrenia. For example, Oertel-Knöchel suggested that altered hemispheric asymmetries could be used as a biomarker for schizophrenia to allow for better identification of at-risk individuals in preclinical stages (Oertel-Knöchel *et al.* 2012).

As already mentioned in several of the preceding sections, one of the core insights of laterality research in schizophrenia patients is the fact that symptom severity seems to be a crucial factor regarding the extent of changes in hemispheric asymmetries (Ocklenburg *et al.* 2015). This has been shown in particular for the link between the experience of auditory verbal hallucinations and changes in language lateralization (Ocklenburg *et al.* 2013). Hugdahl and co-workers put forward a mechanistic model to explain this relationship (Hugdahl *et al.* 2007). They assume that auditory verbal hallucinations are internally generated speech perceptions. As such, they lead to activation of left temporal brain regions, particularly in the peri-Sylvian region. If hallucinating patients are then asked to perform a language-processing task, they fail to show the typical leftward asymmetry as leftward brain regions are already active with generating the hallucinations and thus cannot properly perform the task. Schizophrenia is a highly heterogeneous disorder. Moreover, there is a multitude of hemispheric asymmetries. Therefore, the approach by Hugdahl *et al.* (2007) to map specific laterality alterations to the severity of specific schizophrenia symptoms seems to be more viable than just assuming a general link between schizophrenia as a diagnosis and altered hemispheric asymmetries in all or several cognitive domains. Future studies should use this approach to also investigate other forms of hemispheric asymmetries than language lateralization.

Comparative research

Schizophrenia is highly complex and heterogeneous and while animal models have been developed to investigate specific aspects of the disorder (Jones *et al.* 2011), the use of such models in laterality research is still in its infancy. While the usefulness of animal models for understanding laterality changes in schizophrenia had already been discussed in the 1990s (Cowell *et al.* 1999), only very few empirical studies have been published in this field. One study investigated expression asymmetries in the cortical NMDA receptor-nitric oxide synthase pathway in the Nogo-A-deficient rat model for schizophrenia (Krištofiková *et al.* 2013) and found several changes in expression laterality that corresponded to findings in human patients, for example, abnormal frontoparietal cortical interactions.

Conclusion

Taken together, there is strong evidence for altered hemispheric asymmetries in patients diagnosed with schizophrenia. Compared to healthy controls, they have a higher prevalence of non-right-handedness, show less leftward functional language lateralization, and also show alterations in other forms of functional hemispheric asymmetries. Moreover, patients with schizophrenia show changes in grey and white matter structural asymmetries, such as in the planum temporale or the arcuate fasciculus. Importantly, higher symptom severity has been linked to greater changes in functional hemispheric asymmetries. In general, insights from laterality research can generate new and relevant information about the disrupted brain functioning in schizophrenia and therefore should be included more frequently in research projects on schizophrenia.

Affective disorders

Definition of the disorders

Depression, the most widely acknowledged form of affective disorder, was first described by the Greek physician Hippocrates by introducing the term, melancholia (Lewis 1934). Nowadays, several pathological changes in affect are recognized as mental disorders. Importantly, several core processes disturbed in affective disorders, such as self-perception and emotion processing, show hemispheric asymmetries (Ocklenburg and Güntürkün 2018).

Affective disorders are characterized by disturbances in affect. There are two main types of affective disorders: Depressive disorders such as major depressive disorder (MDD), and bipolar disorder (BD) and related disorders. Major symptoms of depressive episodes are the feeling of worthlessness, reduced self-esteem, and self-confidence, loss of pleasure, motivation, energy and interest, disturbed sleep, loss of appetite, and libido which must be present for at least two weeks (American Psychiatric Association 2013). There are multiple different kinds of affective disorders, mainly differentially diagnosed by the severity of depressive symptoms and frequency of remission as well as the intensity of manic episodes (for BD) (American Psychiatric Association 2013).

The global prevalence for developing MDD is 6–18% (around 264 million people worldwide), with more women being affected than men (Drevets and Furey 2009; WHO 2019). It is categorized into early and late-onset depression. Early-onset depression is characterized by a symptom onset before the age of 40. For late-onset depression, depressive symptoms develop after the age of 40 (Drevets and Furey 2009). In general, MDD usually develops in adulthood, whereas BD tends to develop in adolescence. Multiple genetic factors (Mullins and Lewis 2017; Gordovez and McMahon 2020), as well as environmental influences such as stress, increase the risk for affective disorders (Ding and Dai 2019).

Severe affective disorders usually require pharmacotherapy, such as serotonin reuptake inhibitors (SSRIs) which inhibit the reuptake of the neurotransmitter serotonin into the synapses, (Hohagen and Voderholzer 2019) besides adequate psychotherapeutic intervention. As serotonin is a modulatory transmitter modulating actions of other neurotransmitters, it takes a rather long time (around two weeks) before drugs affect symptoms.

Supportive treatment options can include sleep deprivation, light therapy, electroconvulsive therapy, and deep brain stimulation (Hohagen and Voderholzer 2019). Bipolar disorder is usually treated with mood stabilizers like lithium and/or atypical antipsychotics to treat manic episodes. Both affective disorders profit greatly from (combined) psychotherapy, mainly cognitive behavioural therapy (Hohagen and Voderholzer 2019).

Given the high prevalence of affective disorders and the fact that hemispheric asymmetries in emotion processing are among the most widely investigated forms of laterality, it comes as no surprise that a considerable number of papers on atypical hemispheric asymmetries in affective disorders have been published.

Handedness

The empirical evidence for a higher prevalence of non-right-handedness in affective disorders is mixed. A study in 692 children aged between 4 and 18 years old found that left-handed children had 53% increased odds of suffering from depression compared to right-handed children (Logue *et al.* 2015). However, empirical evidence is less clear in adults. For example, a Canadian study using the Beck Depression Inventory (BDI) in a sample of 541 undergraduate students found that left-handed males showed significantly higher BDI scores than right-handed males or females but did not observe any effects in female participants (Elias *et al.* 2001). Moreover, a smaller study from the 1980s reported that all of the 52 depressed patients tested in the study were strongly right-handed (Moscovitch *et al.* 1981). It was also reported that patients with cyclothymic, hyperthymic, or irritable temperaments show a significantly higher prevalence of non-right-handedness (42%) than patients with depression (24%) (Fasmer *et al.* 2008). The largest study on depression and handedness so far (Denny 2009) used a population survey from 12 European countries (*N*=27482) and reported that left-handers were significantly more likely to have experienced depressive symptoms than right-handers. Altogether, it is clear that meta-analytic integration is needed before any conclusions on handedness in depression can be drawn.

Psychophysiological paradigms

Several authors have investigated language lateralization in patients suffering from affective disorders using the dichotic listening task; the results have been summarized in two review articles (Bruder *et al.* 2017; Gadea *et al.* 2011). In general, results are fairly inconsistent. For example, one study (Wale and Carr 1990) found that the control group showed a typical REA, while depressed subjects did not show an REA, implicating more symmetrical language processing. A later study, however, found that both depressed patients and controls showed an REA with no impairment in the patients compared to controls (Hugdahl *et al.* 2003). To further complicate things, some studies also reported a greater REA in melancholic patients with depression than in controls (Bruder *et al.* 1989). Thus, there is no clear pattern of results regarding verbal dichotic listening performance in depression, and studies in larger samples as well as meta-analytic integration are needed to determine if and how dichotic listening performance is affected by depression.

Functional hemispheric asymmetries in electrophysiological activity

The most widely investigated form of hemispheric asymmetries in patients with affective disorders is probably EEG alpha asymmetries. In general, frontal EEG alpha activity is seen as a marker for the absence of concentrated cognitive activity, so that a leftward EEG alpha asymmetry indicates a rightward asymmetry in cognitive activity and vice versa. This phenomenon has been investigated extensively in the context of emotion processing and psychopathology, following the premise that a rightward frontal alpha asymmetry/leftward brain activity asymmetry is associated with approach and or positive emotions, while leftward frontal alpha asymmetry/rightward brain activity asymmetry is related to avoidance and/or negative emotions (Reznik and Allen 2018). It has been assumed that depressive patients show less activity in left than right frontal sites compared to controls (Bruder *et al.* 2017). This left frontal hypoactivation/higher leftward alpha asymmetry in depressed individuals has been reported in several empirical studies (Debener *et al.* 2000; Henriques and Davidson 1991; Kano *et al.* 1992; Roemer *et al.* 1992; Saletu *et al.* 1996) and has been reviewed extensively elsewhere (Reznik and Allen 2018). However, there also have been findings that were inconsistent with this idea (Blackhart *et al.* 2006; McFarland *et al.* 2006), highlighting the need for meta-analytic integration.

A first meta-analysis found significant effects with moderate effect sizes for both adult (d = 0.54) and infant depression cohorts (d = 0.61), indicating that depression was indeed associated with reduced left frontal and/or increased right frontal brain activity (Thibodeau *et al.* 2006). However, a funnel plot analysis revealed systematic publication bias in favour of significant results in this study, and the authors warned that this issue might have inflated the reported effect sizes.

More than a decade later, a second meta-analysis was performed on data from adult depressive patients. In this study, data from 16 studies including

1883 patients with MDD and 2161 controls were integrated (van der Vinne *et al.* 2017). The results were strikingly different from the earlier meta-analysis. In this study, the authors overall found a non-significant effect with an effect size approaching zero (d = -0.007), indicating that there were no significant differences in frontal EEG alpha asymmetry between depressive patients and controls. The authors also noticed that all studies with a sample size larger than 200 participants approached an effect size of zero, making it highly likely that the significant results of the earlier meta-analysis were mainly driven by inflated effect sizes obtained in small sample studies. This highlights the importance of well-powered studies in laterality research. The authors also highlight that there is a high degree of heterogeneity in studies on alpha asymmetry in depression, making frontal alpha asymmetry an unreliable marker of psychopathology.

A meta-analysis of frontal EEG alpha asymmetries in children integrating 38 studies (Peltola *et al.* 2014) also yielded results that were less clear-cut than those reported by Thibodeau *et al.* (2006). While the authors found a significant association between psychosocial risk to develop depression and greater right frontal asymmetry (d = 0.36), both the association between right frontal asymmetry and internalizing symptoms and the association between left frontal asymmetry and externalizing symptoms failed to reach significance. Taken together, the results of these two more recent meta-analyses suggest that the association between depression and frontal EEG alpha asymmetries might have been overblown by early studies in small sample sizes and that, in fact, the predictive power of EEG asymmetries for depression is low.

Functional hemispheric asymmetries in brain activation

While there are a plethora of functional neuroimaging studies in depressive patients, there have been a surprisingly small number of functional neuroimaging studies specifically investigating hemispheric asymmetries in brain activation in depression. One early fMRI study using an emotional word task reported a rightward asymmetry in the dorsolateral prefrontal cortex in depressed patients compared to controls (Herrington *et al.* 2010). More recently, a functional connectivity study found that patients with MDD showed a rightward asymmetry of functional connectivity of the middle frontal gyrus, orbital middle frontal gyrus, and anterior cingulate gyrus, while healthy controls showed a leftward asymmetry (Ran *et al.* 2020). While both of these studies point towards a right-hemispheric dysfunction in depression, clearly more research is needed in this area of clinical laterality research.

Structural hemispheric asymmetries in grey matter

Older studies with small sample sizes have reported some inconsistent evidence for atypical macrostructural brain asymmetries in patients with affective disorders (Kumar *et al.* 2000; Liu *et al.* 2016). However, the only large-scale study on this topic that has been published so far (De Kovel *et al.* 2019) clearly showed that MDD is not associated with any substantial changes in macrostructural brain asymmetries in grey matter. In this study, the authors analysed 31 separate neuroimaging datasets, resulting in an overall sample size of 2256 patients with MDD and 3503 control subjects. Macrostructural asymmetries (thickness and surface) were analysed for 34 cortical regions. Moreover, macrostructural asymmetries in eight subcortical brain structures were investigated in a slightly larger dataset containing an additional study. No significant group difference was observed, and the largest observed effect had an effect size of Cohen's d = 0.085. Moreover, asymmetries did not show any significant associations with several illness-associated parameters, such as medication use or age of onset. This does, of course, not imply that there are no alterations of structural asymmetries in grey matter at all.

Comparative research

While there is an abundance of studies using animal models to investigate affective disorders, hemispheric asymmetries have only rarely been investigated in a comparative context. One of the few relevant studies investigated how chronic social stress affected cell proliferation in the left and right medial prefrontal cortex (Czéh *et al.* 2007). The authors reported that stressed rats showed a significantly higher rate of cytogenesis in the right medial prefrontal cortex compared to control animals. Interestingly, treatment with fluoxetine, an antidepressant, leads to the abolishment of this hemispheric asymmetry. A more recent study induced depression-like symptoms in rats using a stress protocol and investigated RNA expression asymmetries in the frontotemporal cortex (Farhang *et al.* 2014). Rats were grouped into stress-resistant animals and those that showed anhedonic behaviour. The authors found a rightward expression asymmetry for *Bdnf* in stress-resilient rats. Interestingly, both *Bdnf* and *Ntrk-3* were expressed significantly lower in the right hemisphere of anhedonic rats than in stress-resilient rats. Thus, both of these studies suggest an association between structure and function of the right hemisphere and the pathophysiology of depression. However, due to the very small number of studies, it is clear that more comparative research on hemispheric asymmetries in affective disorders is needed before any conclusions can be drawn.

Conclusion

Taken together, the findings of altered hemispheric asymmetries in affective disorders are considerably less conclusive than what has been found in schizophrenia. Importantly, structural hemispheric asymmetries do not seem to be altered in affective disorders and the data on handedness and verbal dichotic listening are largely unclear. While a substantial number of early EEG studies provided evidence for greater functional activation of the right hemisphere in depressed patients, more recent meta-analyses showed that these effects might have been driven by publication bias and small study bias and that in fact, EEG alpha asymmetries do not show a relation with depression. Thus, in contrast to schizophrenia, there is no strong evidence for altered hemispheric asymmetries in affective disorders. This finding might be somewhat driven by the fact that the prevalence of affective disorders is much higher than that of schizophrenia, potentially leading to higher heterogeneity in these patients than in patients suffering from schizophrenia.

Substance-related and addictive disorders

Definition of the disorders

Substance-related and addictive disorders are characterized by the compulsive use of a substance or compulsive need for a behaviour despite its harmful consequences. Substance-related and addictive disorders can be categorized into two main classes: Substance-related addiction which includes ten different classes of drugs, and non-substance-related addiction such as gambling. They have an intense activation of the reward system in common that leads to a neglect of normal everyday activities (American Psychiatric Association 2013). The symptoms of addiction further include being unable to reduce or quit using, craving, continued use despite social or health problems caused by use, developing tolerance, and spending a great deal of time obtaining the substance, using it, or recovering from its effects (American Psychiatric Association 2013).

In 2015, the estimated prevalence of substance-related addictive disorders among adults was around 15% for heavy alcohol use and daily tobacco smoking and less than 4% for other illicit drugs, with European countries having the highest rates (Peacock *et al.* 2018). Worldwide, approximately 5% of the adult population suffers from substance use disorders, with alcohol and tobacco smoking being the most prevalent, and illicit drugs constituting fewer percentages (Gowing *et al.* 2015). Adolescents are at greater risk as they are experiencing neurodevelopmental changes, especially in the reward circuitry, which makes them more vulnerable to addictive behaviour (Hammond *et al.* 2014). Repeated drug abuse (or exposure to an addictive stimulus in the case of gambling) leads to molecular adaptations in reward processing brain regions which are then mediating addictive behaviour in vulnerable individuals (Nestler 2013). Genetic risk variants increase one's vulnerability as do environmental factors, such as peer pressure (Vink 2016). Substance-related and addictive disorders are thought to be polygenetic with different genetic variants responsible for different types (e.g. substances) of addiction (Hancock *et al.* 2018). So far, treatment options consist of a combination of cognitive behavioural therapy and medication, mostly to treat physical symptoms of withdrawal and craving depending on the substance used (Hohagen and Voderholzer 2019). Research into the origin and pathogenesis of addictive disorders is still small compared to other disorders. However, some studies have already investigated atypical lateralization, mostly studying alcohol addiction.

Handedness and other motor preferences

For drinking behaviour, a large-scale European study with 27,428 participants found that left-handers consume alcohol significantly more often than right-handers (Denny 2011). Moreover, a study that investigated side biases for hands, feet, eyes, and ears in alcoholics, heroin addicts, and healthy controls (Mandal *et al.* 2000) found that alcoholics exhibited a significant reduction of right-side bias for all four forms of laterality. Heroin addicts, however, did not show any atypical laterality. Elevated rates of left-handedness in alcoholics and individuals with risky drinking behaviour were reported by other studies (McNamara *et al.* 1994; Sperling *et al.* 2000). However, a Finnish study on risk factors for alcohol use disorder did not report any significant association with handedness (Poikolainen 2000). For the use of illicit drugs, an Italian study with 1004 participants reported that left-handers had significantly higher rates of lifetime experimentation with heroin, amphetamines, and hallucinogens, but not alcohol or tobacco (Preti *et al.* 2012). This behaviour does, however, not necessarily lead to addiction, and as mentioned, a previous study did not find any evidence for elevated rates of left-handedness in heroin addicts (Mandal *et al.* 2000). Last, a study on social media addiction reported that left-handers show higher rates of pathological social media use (Bouna-Pyrrou *et al.* 2015). Taken together, the evidence for elevated rates of non-right-handedness in addiction is somewhat mixed. More research and a comprehensive meta-analysis of published empirical studies are needed.

Psychophysiological paradigms

While several dichotic listening studies in patients with alcohol use disorder have been published, only one was specifically aimed at analysing hemispheric asymmetries and not general error rates (Drake *et al.* 1990). Here, the authors found that male patients suffering from alcohol use disorder showed a larger REA than healthy controls. They also showed a decreased LEA in a musical dichotic listening task compared to healthy controls. The authors interpreted this finding as an indicator of a specific right-hemispheric dysfunction in alcohol use disorder.

Functional hemispheric asymmetries in electrophysiological activity

Very few studies have investigated EEG measures of hemispheric asymmetries in patients with addiction disorders. One study on frontal alpha band asymmetries found that alcoholic patients showed more right- than left-hemispheric frontal activation, as indicated by a leftward alpha asymmetry (Hayden *et al.* 2006). This finding is comparable to what has been found by some authors for patients suffering from affective disorders, for example, higher left frontal alpha power and therefore higher right frontal brain activation (Henriques and Davidson 1990). However, another study found that cocaine-preferring polysubstance abusers showed altered EEG asymmetries in frontal delta, theta, and alpha power with more rightward lateralization than healthy controls (Roemer *et al.* 1995). This is in contrast to the study by Hayden *et al.* (2006), as the rightward alpha band asymmetry indicated higher leftward brain activation. Clearly, more research is needed in this field before any conclusion can be drawn.

Functional hemispheric asymmetries in brain activation

To our knowledge, only one study has investigated functional neuroimaging of hemispheric asymmetries in patients with addiction disorders so far. In this study, alcoholic patients and healthy controls were tested with two types of memory encoding tasks (word and face encoding) while fMRI was recorded (Yoon *et al.* 2009). The authors did not find any significant differences in brain activity between patients and controls for the left hemisphere-driven language task. In contrast, healthy controls showed rightward lateralization of parahippocampal activity during face encoding that was absent in sufferers of alcohol use disorder. The authors interpreted this finding as evidence for a higher vulnerability of the right hemisphere to alcohol-related damage.

Structural hemispheric asymmetries in grey matter

A few studies have reported altered structural hemispheric asymmetries in grey matter in addiction disorders. For example, one study found that compared to healthy controls, adolescent alcohol users showed reduced left hippocampal volume and more rightward hippocampal asymmetry (Medina *et al*. 2007). However, the third group of adolescents that used both alcohol and marijuana did not differ from the control group, a somewhat puzzling finding that might be explained by the low sample size and resulting low statistical power (16 alcohol users, 26 marijuana and alcohol users, and 21 healthy controls). Another small study (20 patients with alcohol use disorder and 20 healthy controls) reported reduced hemispheric asymmetries of surface shape in the insula (Jung *et al*. 2007). More recently, a voxel-based morphometry study in 19 patients with alcohol use disorder and 20 healthy controls reported increased rightward asymmetries in parts of the cerebellum and the lingual gyrus in patients compared to controls (Zhu *et al*. 2018). Taken together, the three studies on structural hemispheric asymmetries in addiction disorder all have small sample sizes, which might explain the diverging results. More research in larger cohorts is needed before any final conclusions can be drawn.

Structural hemispheric asymmetries in white matter

So far, there is only one diffusion tensor imaging (DTI) study that specifically assessed hemispheric asymmetries in white matter in alcoholic patients compared to healthy controls (Schulte *et al*. 2010). Here, the authors found degraded left posterior cingulate and posterior callosal fibres in patients with chronic alcohol use disorder compared to controls, which somewhat contrasts the idea that it is particularly the right hemisphere that is prone to alcohol-related damage.

Conclusion

Taken together, research on hemispheric asymmetries in patients suffering from substance-related and addictive disorders is still rare and the existing research often seems to have low statistical power. Also, the existing data is often inconclusive and contradicting (e.g. some studies find an elevated rate of left-handedness while others do not, or some studies support the idea of an increased proneness of the right hemisphere to alcohol-related damage while others do not). The field clearly needs large-scale replication studies that are optimally preregistered with clear hypotheses before any deeper understanding of hemispheric asymmetries in substance-related and addictive disorders can be gained. Nevertheless, atypical lateralization in substance-related and addictive disorders is a promising field, as the neurobiology of addiction is well researched and would thus allow for deeper insights into hemispheric dominance in reward processing.

Post traumatic stress disorder

Definition of the disorder

Post traumatic stress disorder (PTSD) develops after exposure to at least one traumatic event or stressor. It is defined by ongoing fear-related reactions whenever re-experiencing (remembering) the event (American Psychiatric Association 2013). PTSD is most typically associated with war but also with natural disasters, mass catastrophes, and sexual abuse (Andreasen 2010). Symptoms include recurring involuntary re-experiencing of the event, avoiding situations, people, or memories that are associated with the event, changes in cognition and mood (regarding the event or oneself), and alterations in arousal and reactivity such as angry outbursts, self-destructing behaviour, and feeling tense (American Psychiatric Association 2013).

The global lifetime prevalence of PTSD is estimated to be around 8% with a 12-month prevalence varying between 1–9% depending on the country (Atwoli *et al.* 2015). Women are two to three times more likely to develop the disorder than men (Olff 2017). A twin study revealed a high genetic risk when being exposed to high-risk trauma events (Sartor *et al.* 2012). In this study, the risk was not specific for PTSD but also for depression. However, family studies regarding the genetics of PTSD are more difficult to conduct as PTSD only develops after experiencing a traumatic event.

PTSD is most effectively treated with behavioural therapy focusing on exposure to the traumatic event leading to acceptance. Another psychological method is eye movement desensitization and reprocessing. Besides, pharmacotherapy can be utilized to treat occurring anxiety or sleep medication to prevent nightmares (Hohagen and Voderholzer 2019). Since stress has been shown to affect both functional and structural hemispheric asymmetries (Ocklenburg *et al.* 2016; Zach *et al.* 2016), it comes as no surprise that several studies have investigated hemispheric asymmetries in patients with PTSD.

Handedness and other motor preferences

Several studies found an association between PTSD and atypical lateral preferences. While one study suggested a link between left-handedness and PTSD (Choudhary and O'carroll 2007) most other studies suggested a link between PTSD and mixed lateral preferences. For example, an early study in 80 PTSD patients and 100 controls (Spivak *et al.* 1998) found that in patients, 70% were right-handed, 7.5% were left-handed, and 22.5% were mixed-handed. In healthy controls, 86% were right-handed, 6% were left-handed, and 8% were mixed-handed. The difference in mixed-handedness between the two groups was significant. Interestingly, a higher prevalence of mixed preferences in PTSD was also found when handedness, footedness, eye dominance, and ear dominance were analysed together. This implies that a more mixed preference pattern in PTSD is not limited to handedness. Later studies in children (Saltzman *et al.* 2006) and adults (Boscarino and Hoffman 2007; Chemtob and Taylor 2003; Ritov and Barnetz 2014) confirmed the general pattern of an increase of mixed lateral preferences in PTSD, making this a well-replicated finding. In a recent book chapter (Ritov and Barnetz 2016), the authors highlighted that this pattern of results can be viewed from two different perspectives. The first perspective assumes that mixed lateral preferences develop before the trauma and therefore represent a risk factor to develop PTSD. The second perspective assumes that exposure to traumatic events could change hemispheric asymmetries, which would be reflected by changes in handedness. There is empirical evidence supporting both ideas, pointing towards a need for longitudinal studies on the subject to properly differentiate between the two theoretical accounts.

Psychophysiological paradigms

Two studies have used the dichotic listening paradigm to assess language lateralization in PTSD. One study in 22 PTSD patients and 23 controls (Asbjørnsen 2011) found that PTSD patients show a stronger REA than controls due to impaired left-ear reporting. Moreover, PTSD patients also showed smaller attention modulation effects than the control group, as reflected by performance in a directed attention condition. The author suggests that this pattern of results reflects an impaired functioning of the right hemisphere in PTSD. A second study (Johnsen *et al.* 2011) also found reduced attention modulation during dichotic listening in PTSD patients as compared to controls. Here, PTSD patients continued to show an REA when instructed to pay attention to the stimuli on the left ear. However, no difference between PTSD patients and controls was observed in the non-forced condition. Thus, more research using the dichotic listening task is needed in PTSD patients before any final conclusions can be drawn.

Functional hemispheric asymmetries in electrophysiological activity

EEG findings on hemispheric asymmetries in PTSD patients are somewhat inconclusive. For example, one study in 14 PTSD patients and 15 healthy controls found a positive correlation between symptom severity in PTSD and rightward frontal asymmetry (Kemp *et al.* 2010). Moreover, a study in female Vietnam War nurse veterans found that PTSD-related arousal symptoms were associated with increased activation of the right parietal lobe (Metzger *et al.* 2004). In contrast, a larger study that compared EEG alpha resting-state asymmetries in 48 PTSD patients to a large normative sample of 1908 healthy controls did not find any significant difference between PTSD patients and controls (Gordon *et al.* 2010). In light of this and further evidence, a recent review article on the topic concluded that resting-state frontal EEG alpha asymmetry has little predictive value for PTSD (Meyer *et al.* 2015). Interestingly, newer research suggests that state-dependent changes in frontal asymmetries in response to negative pictures might be a stronger marker for the development of psychopathology after experiencing trauma than resting-state asymmetries (Meyer *et al.* 2018). In this study, trauma victims who did not develop PTSD showed stronger leftward brain activation than individuals with PTSD when watching negative pictures. This suggests that leftward brain activation after the presentation of negative pictures might be a marker of resilience, an interesting finding that deserves further research.

Structural hemispheric asymmetries in grey matter

While we could not identify any functional neuroimaging studies specifically assessing hemispheric asymmetries in brain activation in PTSD patients and controls, there are a substantial number of studies investigating hemispheric asymmetries in brain structure in PTSD. Based on these studies, several meta-analyses assessing alterations of structural asymmetries in PTSD have been published. For example, one meta-analysis integrated the findings of 13 studies with a total of 215 PTSD patients and 325 control subjects focusing on the hippocampus (Smith 2005). Compared to controls, PTSD patients had a 6.9% smaller left-hemispheric and a 6.6% smaller right-hemispheric hippocampus. Both patients and controls had a slightly smaller left hippocampal volume (about 2.1% smaller compared to the right), but there were no significant group differences in hemispheric asymmetries, supporting the idea of a bilateral, rather than asymmetrical, reduction in hippocampal volume in PTSD. More recently, another meta-analysis on brain structural alterations in PTSD was published, this time assessing differences across the whole brain rather than just the hippocampus (Kühn and Gallinat 2013). In this study, nine voxel-based morphometry studies with a total of 319 subjects were integrated. In contrast to the earlier study, the authors found a volume reduction in PTSD only in the left hippocampus. Besides, a second asymmetric volume reduction cluster was found in the left temporal pole and middle temporal gyrus. Also, PTSD-related volume reductions were observed in two clusters with a centre in the midline of the brain: one in the anterior cingulate cortex, and the other in the ventromedial prefrontal cortex. Subsequently, a meta-analysis and systematic review in a much larger sample of 44 articles with 846 PTSD patients, 520 healthy controls, and 624 controls who experienced trauma but did not develop PTSD confirmed the finding of a leftward asymmetric hippocampal volume reduction in PTSD together with bilateral volume reductions in the anterior cingulate cortex and amygdala (O'Doherty *et al.* 2015). A leftward asymmetric hippocampal volume reduction in PTSD was also reported in another meta-analysis comparing PTSD patients to different control groups (Li *et al.* 2014). Thus, taken together, there is a well-replicated volume reduction asymmetry in the hippocampus associated with PTSD. Interestingly, it has been suggested that a reduction of hippocampal volume might be a risk factor to develop PTSD, rather than a consequence of the trauma (Li *et al.* 2014). This idea is mainly based on a study in which twin pairs, one of which had a traumatic combat experience while the other did not, were investigated (Gilbertson *et al.* 2002). In this study, the authors found that patients with PTSD with a smaller total hippocampal volume showed more severe PTSD symptoms. Interestingly, smaller total hippocampal volume in unaffected brothers was significantly correlated with symptom severity in the twin suffering from PTSD. This suggests that hippocampal volume reduction is not exclusively an effect of trauma exposure but that people with a genetic disposition for smaller hippocampal volume might have a greater risk to develop PTSD if they experience trauma.

Structural hemispheric asymmetries in white matter

In addition to changes in structural asymmetries in grey matter, structural asymmetries in white matter structures have been investigated on the meta-analytic level. An early meta-analysis of seven whole-brain DTI studies in adult PTSD patients and controls (Daniels *et al.* 2013) reported both increases and decreases of fractional anisotropy (FA; a marker of white matter structural integrity) in PTSD patients compared to controls. In this study, activation-likelihood (ALE) meta-analysis was used, even though seven studies may be too few to generate reliable results; it has been recommended that at least 20 different experiments be included in ALE meta-analysis to have sufficient statistical power to detect moderate effects (Eickhoff *et al.* 2016). The authors reported FA decreases in several white matter structures, with the strongest effects being found for a cluster in the right cingulum followed by a cluster in the left cingulum. Surprisingly, FA increases in PTSD patients compared to controls were found in bilateral clusters in the left and right cingulum as well as in the left and right superior longitudinal fasciculus. Thus, the cingulum should both decrease and increase in FA in patients in this study. However, the findings from the small meta-analysis were not replicated in the largest study on white matter changes in PTSD so far. This study was conducted by the PGC-ENIGMA PTSD consortium and integrated white matter data across the whole brain in 1426 patients with PTSD and 1621 controls from 28 cohorts (Dennis *et al*. 2019). In this study, PTSD patients showed significantly lower FA in the tapetum segment of the corpus callosum compared to controls. While the effect was present in both the left and the right tapetum, it had a substantially larger effect size for the left tapetum. The tapetum is the subsegment of the corpus callosum that connects parts of the two temporal lobes, in particular the two hippocampi. Thus, these findings suggest that structural connectivity between the two hippocampi is disturbed in PTSD.

Conclusion

Taken together, research on altered hemispheric asymmetries in PTSD has revealed two well-replicated findings. On the one hand, there is an association of PTSD with a higher prevalence of mixed-handedness on the behavioural level. On the other hand, there is a leftward asymmetry of hippocampal volume reduction and callosal connections between the two hippocampi. Other fields of laterality research, such as EEG experiments and the dichotic listening task, have yielded results which are less clear and thus deserve more investigation in future studies.

References

Abdul-Rahman, M.F., *et al*., 2012. Arcuate fasciculus abnormalities and their relationship with psychotic symptoms in schizophrenia. *PLoS One*, 7 (1), e29315.

Agcaoglu, O., *et al*., 2018. Decreased hemispheric connectivity and decreased intra- and inter- hemisphere asymmetry of resting state functional network connectivity in schizophrenia. *Brain Imaging and Behavior*, 12 (3), 615–630.

Alary, M., *et al*., 2013. Functional hemispheric lateralization for language in patients with schizophrenia. *Schizophrenia Research*, 149 (1–3), 42–47.

American Psychiatric Association, 2013. *Diagnostic and statistical manual of mental disorders. DSM-5*. 5th ed. Washington, DC: American Psychiatric Publishing.

Andreasen, N.C., 2010. Posttraumatic stress disorder: a history and a critique. *Annals of the New York Academy of Sciences*, 1208, 67–71.

Artiges, E., *et al*., 2000. Altered hemispheric functional dominance during word generation in negative schizophrenia. *Schizophrenia Bulletin*, 26 (3), 709–721.

Asbjørnsen, A.E., 2011. Dichotic listening performance suggests right hemisphere involvement in PTSD. *Laterality*, 16 (4), 401–422.

Atwoli, L., *et al*., 2015. Epidemiology of posttraumatic stress disorder: prevalence, correlates and consequences. *Current Opinion in Psychiatry*, 28 (4), 307–311.

Barry, S.J.E., Gaughan, T.M., and Hunter, R., 2012. Schizophrenia. *BMJ Clinical Evidence*, 2012.

Blackhart, G.C., Minnix, J.A., and Kline, J.P., 2006. Can EEG asymmetry patterns predict future development of anxiety and depression? A preliminary study. *Biological Psychology*, 72 (1), 46–50.

Bleich-Cohen, M., *et al.*, 2012. Diminished language lateralization in schizophrenia corresponds to impaired inter-hemispheric functional connectivity. *Schizophrenia Research*, 134 (2–3), 131–136.

Bleuler, E., 1908. Die Prognose der Dementia praecox (Schizophreniegruppe). *Allgemeine Zeitschrift für Psychiatrie und psychisch-gerichtliche Medizin*, 65, 436–480.

Boscarino, J.A., and Hoffman, S.N., 2007. Consistent association between mixed lateral preference and PTSD: confirmation among a national study of 2490 US Army Vietnam veterans. *Psychosomatic Medicine*, 69 (4), 365–369.

Bouna-Pyrrou, P., *et al.*, 2015. Internet gaming disorder, social network disorder and laterality: handedness relates to pathological use of social networks. *Journal of Neural Transmission (Vienna, Austria: 1996)*, 122 (8), 1187–1196.

Bourne, V.J., 2006. The divided visual field paradigm: methodological considerations. *Laterality*, 11 (4), 373–393.

Bruder, G.E., *et al.*, 1989. Cerebral laterality and depression: differences in perceptual asymmetry among diagnostic subtypes. *Journal of Abnormal Psychology*, 98 (2), 177–186.

Bruder, G.E., Stewart, J.W., and McGrath, P.J., 2017. Right brain, left brain in depressive disorders: clinical and theoretical implications of behavioral, electrophysiological and neuroimaging findings. *Neuroscience and Biobehavioral Reviews*, 78, 178–191.

Cascio, M.T., *et al.*, 2012. Gender and duration of untreated psychosis: a systematic review and meta-analysis. *Early Intervention in Psychiatry*, 6 (2), 115–127.

Chemtob, C.M., and Taylor, K.B., 2003. Mixed lateral preference and parental left-handedness: possible markers of risk for PTSD. *The Journal of Nervous and Mental Disease*, 191 (5), 332–338.

Choudhary, C.J., and O'Carroll, R.E., 2007. Left hand preference is related to post-traumatic stress disorder. *Journal of Traumatic Stress*, 20 (3), 365–369.

Coan, J.A., and Allen, J.J.B., 2004. Frontal EEG asymmetry as a moderator and mediator of emotion. *Biological Psychology*, 67 (1–2), 7–49.

Cowell, P.E., Fitch, R.H., and Denenberg, V.H., 1999. Laterality in animals: relevance to schizophrenia. *Schizophrenia Bulletin*, 25 (1), 41–62.

Crow, T.J., 2008. The 'big bang' theory of the origin of psychosis and the faculty of language. *Schizophrenia Research*, 102 (1–3), 31–52.

Czéh, B., *et al.*, 2007. Chronic social stress inhibits cell proliferation in the adult medial prefrontal cortex: hemispheric asymmetry and reversal by fluoxetine treatment. *Neuropsychopharmacology: Official Publication of the American College of Neuropsychopharmacology*, 32 (7), 1490–1503.

Daniels, J.K., *et al.*, 2013. White matter integrity and its relationship to PTSD and childhood trauma—a systematic review and meta-analysis. *Depression and Anxiety*, 30 (3), 207–216.

Debener, S., *et al.*, 2000. Is resting anterior EEG alpha asymmetry a trait marker for depression? Findings for healthy adults and clinically depressed patients. *Neuropsychobiology*, 41 (1), 31–37.

De Kovel, C.G.F., *et al.*, 2019. No alterations of brain structural asymmetry in major depressive disorder: an ENIGMA consortium analysis. *The American Journal of Psychiatry*, 176 (12), 1039–1049.

Dennis, E.L., *et al.*, 2019. Altered white matter microstructural organization in posttraumatic stress disorder across 3047 adults: results from the PGC-ENIGMA PTSD consortium. *Molecular Psychiatry*, Online ahead of print. https://www.nature.com/articles/s41380-019-0631-x#citeas.

Denny, K., 2009. Handedness and depression: evidence from a large population survey. *Laterality*, 14 (3), 246–255.

Denny, K., 2011. Handedness and drinking behaviour. *British Journal of Health Psychology*, 16 (Pt 2), 386–395.

Ding, Y., and Dai, J., 2019. Advance in stress for depressive disorder. *In:* Y. Fang, ed. *Depressive disorders: mechanisms, measurement and management.* Singapore: Springer, 147–178.

Dollfus, S., *et al.*, 2005. Atypical hemispheric specialization for language in right-handed schizophrenia patients. *Biological Psychiatry*, 57 (9), 1020–1028.

Dragovic, M., and Hammond, G., 2005. Handedness in schizophrenia: a quantitative review of evidence. *Acta Psychiatrica Scandinavica*, 111 (6), 410–419.

Drake, A.I., Hannay, H.J., and Gam, J., 1990. Effects of chronic alcoholism on hemispheric functioning: an examination of gender differences for cognitive and dichotic listening tasks. *Journal of Clinical and Experimental Neuropsychology*, 12 (5), 781–797.

Drevets, W.C., and Furey, M.L., 2009. Depression and the brain. *In:* L.R. Squire, ed. *Encyclopedia of neuroscience.* Amsterdam: Elsevier, 459–470.

Eickhoff, S.B., *et al.*, 2016. Behavior, sensitivity, and power of activation likelihood estimation characterized by massive empirical simulation. *NeuroImage*, 137, 70–85.

Elert, E., 2014. Aetiology: searching for schizophrenia's roots. *Nature*, 508 (7494), S2–S3.

Elias, L.J., Saucier, D.M., and Guylee, M.J., 2001. Handedness and depression in university students: a sex by handedness interaction. *Brain and Cognition*, 46 (1–2), 125–129.

Eranti, S.V., *et al.*, 2013. Gender difference in age at onset of schizophrenia: a meta-analysis. *Psychological Medicine*, 43 (1), 155–167.

Farhang, S., *et al.*, 2014. Asymmetrical expression of BDNF and NTRK3 genes in frontoparietal cortex of stress-resilient rats in an animal model of depression. *Synapse (New York, N.Y.)*, 68 (9), 387–393.

Fasmer, O.B., *et al.*, 2008. Non-right-handedness is associated with migraine and soft bipolarity in patients with mood disorders. *Journal of Affective Disorders*, 108 (3), 217–224.

Flor-Henry, P., 1969. Psychosis and temporal lobe epilepsy. A controlled investigation. *Epilepsia*, 10 (3), 363–395.

Gadea, M., *et al.*, 2011. The sad, the angry, and the asymmetrical brain: dichotic listening studies of negative affect and depression. *Brain and Cognition*, 76 (2), 294–299.

Geoffroy, P.A., *et al.*, 2014. The Arcuate Fasciculus in auditory-verbal hallucinations: a meta-analysis of diffusion-tensor-imaging studies. *Schizophrenia Research*, 159 (1), 234–237.

Gilbertson, M.W., *et al.*, 2002. Smaller hippocampal volume predicts pathologic vulnerability to psychological trauma. *Nature Neuroscience*, 5 (11), 1242–1247.

Gordon, E., Palmer, D.M., and Cooper, N., 2010. EEG alpha asymmetry in schizophrenia, depression, PTSD, panic disorder, ADHD and conduct disorder. *Clinical EEG and Neuroscience*, 41 (4), 178–183.

Gordovez, F.J.A., and McMahon, F.J., 2020. The genetics of bipolar disorder. *Molecular Psychiatry*, 25, 544–559.

Gowing, L.R., *et al.*, 2015. Global statistics on addictive behaviours: 2014 status report. *Addiction*, 110 (6), 904–919.

Gruzelier, J., 1994. Syndromes of schizophrenia and schizotypy, hemispheric imbalance and sex differences: implications for developmental psychopathology. *International Journal of Psychophysiology: Official Journal of the International Organization of Psychophysiology*, 18 (3), 167–178.

Gruzelier, J., Wilson, L., and Richardson, A., 1999. Cognitive asymmetry patterns in schizophrenia: retest reliability and modification with recovery. *International Journal of Psychophysiology: Official Journal of the International Organization of Psychophysiology*, 34 (3), 323–331.

Hammond, C.J., Mayes, L.C., and Potenza, M.N., 2014. Neurobiology of adolescent substance use and addictive behaviors: treatment implications. *Adolescent Medicine: State of the Art Reviews*, 25 (1), 15–32.

Hancock, D.B., *et al.*, 2018. Human genetics of addiction: new insights and future directions. *Current Psychiatry Reports*, 20 (2), 8.

Hayden, E.P., *et al.*, 2006. Patterns of regional brain activity in alcohol-dependent subjects. *Alcoholism, Clinical and Experimental Research*, 30 (12), 1986–1991.

Health Quality Ontario, 2018. Cognitive behavioural therapy for psychosis: a health technology assessment. *Ontario Health Technology Assessment Series*, 18 (5), 1–141.

Henriques, J.B., and Davidson, R.J., 1990. Regional brain electrical asymmetries discriminate between previously depressed and healthy control subjects. *Journal of Abnormal Psychology*, 99 (1), 22–31.

Henriques, J.B., and Davidson, R.J., 1991. Left frontal hypoactivation in depression. *Journal of Abnormal Psychology*, 100 (4), 535–545.

Herrington, J.D., *et al.*, 2010. Localization of asymmetric brain function in emotion and depression. *Psychophysiology*, 47 (3), 442–454.

Hirnstein, M., and Hugdahl, K., 2014. Excess of non-right-handedness in schizophrenia: meta-analysis of gender effects and potential biases in handedness assessment. *The British Journal of Psychiatry: The Journal of Mental Science*, 205 (4), 260–267.

Hohagen, F., and Voderholzer, U., eds., 2019. *Therapie psychischer Erkrankungen. State of the art*. 14th ed. München, Deutschland: Elsevier.

Hugdahl, K., 2000. Lateralization of cognitive processes in the brain. *Acta Psychologica*, 105 (2–3), 211–235.

Hugdahl, K., *et al.*, 2003. Attentional and executive dysfunctions in schizophrenia and depression: evidence from dichotic listening performance. *Biological Psychiatry*, 53 (7), 609–616.

Hugdahl, K., *et al.*, 2007. Auditory hallucinations in schizophrenia: the role of cognitive, brain structural and genetic disturbances in the left temporal lobe. *Frontiers in Human Neuroscience*, 1, 6.

Insel, T.R., 2010. Rethinking schizophrenia. *Nature*, 468 (7321), 187–193.

Jalili, M., *et al.*, 2010. Attenuated asymmetry of functional connectivity in schizophrenia: a high-resolution EEG study. *Psychophysiology*, 47 (4), 706–716.

Johnsen, G.E., Kanagaratnam, P., and Asbjørnsen, A.E., 2011. Patients with posttraumatic stress disorder show decreased cognitive control: evidence from dichotic listening. *Journal of the International Neuropsychological Society: JINS*, 17 (2), 344–353.

Jones, C.A., Watson, D.J.G., and Fone, K.C.F., 2011. Animal models of schizophrenia. *British Journal of Pharmacology*, 164 (4), 1162–1194.

Jung, Y.C., *et al.*, 2007. Shape deformation of the insula in alcoholics: reduction of left-right asymmetry. *Neuroreport*, 18 (17), 1787–1791.

Kano, K., *et al.*, 1992. The topographical features of EEGs in patients with affective disorders. *Electroencephalography and Clinical Neurophysiology*, 83 (2), 124–129.

Ke, M., *et al.*, 2010. Bilateral functional asymmetry disparity in positive and negative schizophrenia revealed by resting-state fMRI. *Psychiatry Research*, 182 (1), 30–39.

Kemp, A.H., *et al.*, 2010. Disorder specificity despite comorbidity: resting EEG alpha asymmetry in major depressive disorder and post-traumatic stress disorder. *Biological Psychology*, 85 (2), 350–354.

Krištofiková, Z., *et al.*, 2013. N-Methyl-d-aspartate receptor—nitric oxide synthase pathway in the cortex of Nogo-A-deficient rats in relation to brain laterality and schizophrenia. *Frontiers in Behavioral Neuroscience*, 7, 90.

Kubicki, M., *et al.*, 2002. Uncinate fasciculus findings in schizophrenia: a magnetic resonance diffusion tensor imaging study. *The American Journal of Psychiatry*, 159 (5), 813–820.

Kühn, S., and Gallinat, J., 2013. Gray matter correlates of posttraumatic stress disorder: a quantitative meta-analysis. *Biological Psychiatry*, 73 (1), 70–74.

Kumar, A., *et al.*, 2000. Volumetric asymmetries in late-onset mood disorders: an attenuation of frontal asymmetry with depression severity. *Psychiatry Research: Neuroimaging*, 100 (1), 41–47.

Leach, E.L., *et al.*, 2014. The imprinted gene LRRTM1 mediates schizotypy and handedness in a nonclinical population. *Journal of Human Genetics*, 59 (6), 332–336.

Lenzenweger, M.F., 2018. Schizotypy, schizotypic psychopathology and schizophrenia. *World Psychiatry: Official Journal of the World Psychiatric Association (WPA)*, 17 (1), 25–26.

Lewis, A.J., 1934. Melancholia: a historical review. *Journal of Mental Science*, 80 (328), 1–42.

Li, L., *et al.*, 2014. Grey matter reduction associated with posttraumatic stress disorder and traumatic stress. *Neuroscience and Biobehavioral Reviews*, 43, 163–172.

Liu, W., *et al.*, 2016. Structural asymmetry of dorsolateral prefrontal cortex correlates with depressive symptoms: evidence from healthy individuals and patients with major depressive disorder. *Neuroscience Bulletin*, 32 (3), 217–226.

Løberg, E.-M., Jørgensen, H.A., and Hugdahl, K., 2002. Functional brain asymmetry and attentional modulation in young and stabilised schizophrenic patients: a dichotic listening study. *Psychiatry Research*, 109 (3), 281–287.

Logue, D.D., *et al.*, 2015. Psychiatric disorders and left-handedness in children living in an urban environment. *Laterality*, 20 (2), 249–256.

Mandal, M.K., *et al.*, 2000. Side-bias in alcohol and heroin addicts. *Alcohol and Alcoholism (Oxford, Oxfordshire)*, 35 (4), 381–383.

McFarland, B.R., *et al.*, 2006. Behavioral activation system deficits predict the six-month course of depression. *Journal of Affective Disorders*, 91 (2–3), 229–234.

McNamara, P., *et al.*, 1994. Markers of cerebral lateralization and alcoholism. *Perceptual and Motor Skills*, 79 (3 Pt 2), 1435–1440.

Medina, K.L., *et al.*, 2007. Effects of alcohol and combined marijuana and alcohol use during adolescence on hippocampal volume and asymmetry. *Neurotoxicology and Teratology*, 29 (1), 141–152.

Metzger, L.J., *et al.*, 2004. PTSD arousal and depression symptoms associated with increased right-sided parietal EEG asymmetry. *Journal of Abnormal Psychology*, 113 (2), 324–329.

Meyer, T., *et al.*, 2015. The role of frontal EEG asymmetry in post-traumatic stress disorder. *Biological Psychology*, 108, 62–77.

Meyer, T., *et al.*, 2018. Frontal EEG asymmetry during symptom provocation predicts subjective responses to intrusions in survivors with and without PTSD. *Psychophysiology*, 55 (1).

Min, S.K., and Oh, B.H., 1992. Hemispheric asymmetry in visual recognition of words and motor response in schizophrenic and depressive patients. *Biological Psychiatry*, 31 (3), 255–262.

Moher, D., *et al.*, 2009. Preferred reporting items for systematic reviews and meta-analyses: the PRISMA statement. *Annals of Internal Medicine*, 151 (4), 264–269, W64.

Moscovitch, M., Strauss, E., and Olds, J., 1981. Handedness and dichotic listening performance in patients with unipolar endogenous depression who received ECT. *The American Journal of Psychiatry*, 138 (7), 988–990.

Mullins, N., and Lewis, C.M., 2017. Genetics of depression: progress at last. *Current Psychiatry Reports*, 19 (8), 43.

Nestler, E.J., 2013. Cellular basis of memory for addiction. *Dialogues in Clinical Neuroscience*, 15 (4), 431–443.

Ocklenburg, S., *et al.*, 2013. Auditory hallucinations and reduced language lateralization in schizophrenia: a meta-analysis of dichotic listening studies. *Journal of the International Neuropsychological Society: JINS*, 19 (4), 410–418.

Ocklenburg, S., *et al.*, 2015. Laterality and mental disorders in the postgenomic age—a closer look at schizophrenia and language lateralization. *Neuroscience and Biobehavioral Reviews*, 59, 100–110.

Ocklenburg, S., *et al.*, 2016. Stress and laterality—the comparative perspective. *Physiology & Behavior*, 164 (Pt A), 321–329.

Ocklenburg, S., and Güntürkün, O., 2018. *The lateralized brain. The neuroscience and evolution of hemispheric asymmetries.* London: Academic Press.

O'Doherty, D.C.M., *et al.*, 2015. A systematic review and meta-analysis of magnetic resonance imaging measurement of structural volumes in posttraumatic stress disorder. *Psychiatry Research*, 232 (1), 1–33.

Oertel-Knöchel, V., *et al.*, 2010. Reduced laterality as a trait marker of schizophrenia—evidence from structural and functional neuroimaging. *The Journal of Neuroscience: The Official Journal of the Society for Neuroscience*, 30 (6), 2289–2299.

Oertel-Knöchel, V., *et al.*, 2012. Abnormal functional and structural asymmetry as biomarker for schizophrenia. *Current Topics in Medicinal Chemistry*, 12 (21), 2434–2451.

Oertel-Knöchel, V., and Linden, D.E.J., 2011. Cerebral asymmetry in schizophrenia. *The Neuroscientist: A Review Journal Bringing Neurobiology, Neurology and Psychiatry*, 17 (5), 456–467.

Olff, M., 2017. Sex and gender differences in post-traumatic stress disorder: an update. *European Journal of Psychotraumatology*, 8 (Suppl 4), 1351204.

Papadatou-Pastou, M., *et al.*, 2008. Sex differences in left-handedness: a meta-analysis of 144 studies. *Psychological Bulletin*, 134 (5), 677–699.

Parakh, P., and Basu, D., 2013. Cannabis and psychosis: have we found the missing links? *Asian Journal of Psychiatry*, 6 (4), 281–287.

Pardiñas, A.F., *et al.*, 2018. Common schizophrenia alleles are enriched in mutation-intolerant genes and in regions under strong background selection. *Nature Genetics*, 50 (3), 381–389.

Peacock, A., *et al.*, 2018. Global statistics on alcohol, tobacco and illicit drug use: 2017 status report. *Addiction*, 113 (10), 1905–1926.

Peltola, M.J., *et al.*, 2014. Resting frontal EEG asymmetry in children: meta-analyses of the effects of psychosocial risk factors and associations with internalizing and externalizing behavior. *Developmental Psychobiology*, 56 (6), 1377–1389.

Picchioni, M.M., and Murray, R.M., 2007. Schizophrenia. *BMJ (Clinical Research Ed.)*, 335 (7610), 91–95.

Poikolainen, K., 2000. Risk factors for alcohol dependence: a case-control study. *Alcohol and Alcoholism (Oxford, Oxfordshire)*, 35 (2), 190–196.

Preti, A., *et al.*, 2012. Left-handedness is statistically linked to lifetime experimentation with illicit drugs. *Laterality*, 17 (3), 318–339.

Ran, S., *et al.*, 2020. Atrophic corpus callosum associated with altered functional asymmetry in major depressive disorder. *Neuropsychiatric Disease and Treatment*, 16, 1473–1482.

Razafimandimby, A., *et al.*, 2007. Stability of functional language lateralization over time in schizophrenia patients. *Schizophrenia Research*, 94 (1–3), 197–206.

Remington, G., *et al.*, 2017. Guidelines for the pharmacotherapy of schizophrenia in adults. *Canadian Journal of Psychiatry. Revue Canadienne de Psychiatrie*, 62 (9), 604–616.

Reznik, S.J., and Allen, J.J.B., 2018. Frontal asymmetry as a mediator and moderator of emotion: an updated review. *Psychophysiology*, 55 (1).

Ribolsi, M., *et al.*, 2014. Abnormal asymmetry of brain connectivity in schizophrenia. *Frontiers in Human Neuroscience*, 8, 1010.

Ritov, G., and Barnetz, Z., 2014. The interrelationships between moral attitudes, posttraumatic stress disorder symptoms and mixed lateral preference in Israeli reserve combat troops. *The International Journal of Social Psychiatry*, 60 (6), 606–612.

Ritov, G., and Barnetz, Z., 2016. PTSD and lateral preference: overview of the relationship between distress symptoms and handedness. *In: Comprehensive guide to post-traumatic stress disorders*. Cham: Springer, 435–463.

Roemer, R.A., *et al.*, 1992. Quantitative EEG in elderly depressives. *Brain Topography*, 4 (4), 285–290.

Roemer, R.A., *et al.*, 1995. Quantitative electroencephalographic analyses in cocaine-preferring polysubstance abusers during abstinence. *Psychiatry Research*, 58 (3), 247–257.

Saletu, B., *et al.*, 1996. Hormonal, syndromal and EEG mapping studies in menopausal syndrome patients with and without depression as compared with controls. *Maturitas*, 23 (1), 91–105.

Saltzman, K.M., *et al.*, 2006. Mixed lateral preference in posttraumatic stress disorder. *The Journal of Nervous and Mental Disease*, 194 (2), 142–144.

Sartor, C.E., *et al.*, 2012. Common heritable contributions to low-risk trauma, high-risk trauma, posttraumatic stress disorder, and major depression. *Archives of General Psychiatry*, 69 (3), 293–299.

Schizophrenia Working Group of the Psychiatric Genomics Consortium, 2014. Biological insights from 108 schizophrenia-associated genetic loci. *Nature*, 511 (7510), 421–427.

Schulte, T., *et al.*, 2010. White matter fiber degradation attenuates hemispheric asymmetry when integrating visuomotor information. *The Journal of Neuroscience: The Official Journal of the Society for Neuroscience*, 30 (36), 12168–12178.

Shapleske, J., *et al.*, 1999. The planum temporale: a systematic, quantitative review of its structural, functional and clinical significance. *Brain Research. Brain Research Reviews*, 29 (1), 26–49.

Smith, E.E., *et al.*, 2017. Assessing and conceptualizing frontal EEG asymmetry: an updated primer on recording, processing, analyzing, and interpreting frontal alpha asymmetry. *International Journal of Psychophysiology: Official Journal of the International Organization of Psychophysiology*, 111, 98–114.

Smith, M.E., 2005. Bilateral hippocampal volume reduction in adults with posttraumatic stress disorder: a meta-analysis of structural MRI studies. *Hippocampus*, 15 (6), 798–807.

Somers, M., *et al.*, 2009. Hand-preference and population schizotypy: a meta-analysis. *Schizophrenia Research*, 108 (1–3), 25–32.

Sommer, I., *et al.*, 2001a. Handedness, language lateralisation and anatomical asymmetry in schizophrenia: meta-analysis. *The British Journal of Psychiatry: The Journal of Mental Science*, 178, 344–351.

Sommer, I., *et al.*, 2003. Language lateralization in female patients with schizophrenia: an fMRI study. *Schizophrenia Research*, 60 (2–3), 183–190.

Sommer, I., and Kahn, R.S., eds., 2009. *Language lateralization and psychosis*. Cambridge: Cambridge University Press.

Sommer, I., Ramsey, N.F., and Kahn, R.S., 2001b. Language lateralization in schizophrenia, an fMRI study. *Schizophrenia Research*, 52 (1–2), 57–67.

Sperling, W., *et al.*, 2000. The concept of abnormal hemispheric organization in addiction research. *Alcohol and Alcoholism (Oxford, Oxfordshire)*, 35 (4), 394–399.

Spironelli, C., and Angrilli, A., 2015. Language-related gamma EEG frontal reduction is associated with positive symptoms in schizophrenia patients. *Schizophrenia Research*, 165 (1), 22–29.

Spivak, B., *et al.*, 1998. Lateral preference in post-traumatic stress disorder. *Psychological Medicine*, 28 (1), 229–232.

Sun, Y., *et al.*, 2017. Reduced hemispheric asymmetry of brain anatomical networks is linked to schizophrenia: a connectome study. *Cerebral Cortex (New York, N.Y.: 1991)*, 27 (1), 602–615.

Tervaniemi, M., and Hugdahl, K., 2003. Lateralization of auditory-cortex functions. *Brain Research. Brain Research Reviews*, 43 (3), 231–246.

Thibodeau, R., Jorgensen, R.S., and Kim, S., 2006. Depression, anxiety, and resting frontal EEG asymmetry: a meta-analytic review. *Journal of Abnormal Psychology*, 115 (4), 715–729.

Tran, U.S., Stieger, S., and Voracek, M., 2015. Mixed-footedness is a more relevant predictor of schizotypy than mixed-handedness. *Psychiatry Research*, 225 (3), 446–451.

van der Vinne, N., *et al.*, 2017. Frontal alpha asymmetry as a diagnostic marker in depression: fact or fiction? A meta-analysis. *NeuroImage. Clinical*, 16, 79–87.

van Os, J., and Kapur, S., 2009. Schizophrenia. *The Lancet*, 374 (9690), 635–645.

Vink, J.M., 2016. Genetics of addiction: future focus on gene × environment interaction? *Journal of Studies on Alcohol and Drugs*, 77 (5), 684–687.

Wale, J., and Carr, V., 1990. Differences in dichotic listening asymmetries in depression according to symptomatology. *Journal of Affective Disorders*, 18 (1), 1–9.

Weiss, E.M., *et al.*, 2004. Brain activation patterns during a verbal fluency test- a functional MRI study in healthy volunteers and patients with schizophrenia. *Schizophrenia Research*, 70 (2–3), 287–291.

Weiss, E.M., *et al.*, 2006. Language lateralization in unmedicated patients during an acute episode of schizophrenia: a functional MRI study. *Psychiatry Research*, 146 (2), 185–190.

Westerhausen, R., and Kompus, K., 2018. How to get a left-ear advantage: a technical review of assessing brain asymmetry with dichotic listening. *Scandinavian Journal of Psychology*, 59 (1), 66–73.

WHO, 2019. Mental disorders. www.who.int/news-room/fact-sheets/detail/mental-disorders.

Wigan, A.L., 1844. *A new view of insanity: the duality of the mind proved by the structure, functions and diseases of the brain and by the phenomena of mental derangement and shown to be essential to moral responsibility.* London: Longman, Brown, Green, and Longmans.

Xie, W., *et al.*, 2018. Functional brain lateralization in schizophrenia based on the variability of resting-state fMRI signal. *Progress in Neuro-Psychopharmacology & Biological Psychiatry*, 86, 114–121.

Yoon, H.W., *et al.*, 2009. Differential activation of face memory encoding tasks in alcohol-dependent patients compared to healthy subjects: an fMRI study. *Neuroscience Letters*, 450 (3), 311–316.

Zach, P., *et al.*, 2016. Effect of stress on structural brain asymmetry. *Neuro Endocrinology Letters*, 37 (4), 253–264.

Zhu, J., *et al.*, 2018. Abnormal gray matter asymmetry in alcohol dependence. *Neuroreport*, 29 (9), 753–759.

4 Lateralization in neurological disorders

Introduction

Neurological and neurodegenerative disorders such as Parkinson's disease (PD), multiple sclerosis (MS), and Alzheimer's disease (AD) are different from the neurodevelopmental and psychiatric disorders discussed in the previous chapters in many aspects. In most cases, the pathogenesis of neurological disorders on the cellular level is much better understood. Also, there is less evidence for altered functional and structural hemispheric asymmetries in these patient groups than in most of those previously described. There is, however, one important finding that is often neglected in the laterality literature: the role of lesion laterality. Especially for PD, it has been shown that disease severity and experienced symptoms are affected by lesion laterality. In this chapter, we want to highlight these findings while also reviewing the literature on functional and structural hemispheric asymmetries in neurological disorders.

Parkinson's disease

Definition of the disorder

Parkinson's disease (PD) is a progressive neurodegenerative disorder (Kalia and Lang 2015) associated with loss of dopaminergic neurons in the substantia nigra. Symptoms include impaired motor functions leading to slow movements, tremors, rigidity, bradykinesia, and unstable balance (Sveinbjornsdottir 2016). Non-motor impairments such as autonomic and sensory dysfunction and neuropsychiatric symptoms such as dementia or depression can occur as well (Poewe 2008). After AD, PD is the most common neurological disorder worldwide (Wallin *et al.* 2019) with a prevalence of 1% in the population over 60 years of age (Tysnes and Storstein 2017). Parkinson's disease prevalence increases with age, with no sex differences reported (De

Rijk *et al.* 2000). Mutations in more than 20 genes have been associated with PD (Blauwendraat *et al.* 2020). Environmental influences associated with PD include cigarette smoking, alcohol consumption, head injuries, and a lack of physical activity (Bellou *et al.* 2016). PD is usually treated with dopaminergic drugs to reduce motor dysfunctions (Sveinbjornsdottir 2016). At first, patients respond well to Levodopa (L-DOPA), a precursor of dopamine. At the point when dopaminergic neurons can no longer store enough dopamine, other drugs, such as monoamine oxidase blockers or dopamine receptor antagonists, are required. For PD patients with severe symptoms, deep brain electrical stimulation is a treatment option as well (Sveinbjornsdottir 2016).

Lesion laterality

Asymmetry is an inherent characteristic of PD. Typically, PD patients present with asymmetrical motor symptoms, and symptoms usually show a unilateral onset (Agosta *et al.* 2020; Djaldetti *et al.* 2006). A recent study revealed that only 16.4% of PD patients showed symmetrical clinical syndromes (Gómez-Esteban *et al.* 2010), making asymmetry the rule rather than the exception. The asymmetrical onset of PD motor symptoms has been linked to asymmetries in dopamine depletion in the substantia nigra (Kempster *et al.* 1989). Importantly, the side of onset impacts PD symptoms and their severity, and for this reason, PD patients with right-sided motor symptom onset have been compared to patients with left-sided motor symptom onset in several studies (Cronin-Golomb 2010; Verreyt *et al.* 2011). For example, a left-sided onset of motor symptoms has been associated with stronger cognitive decline and more neuropsychological deficits than a right-sided onset of motor symptoms (Riederer and Sian-Hülsmann 2012; Riederer *et al.* 2018). Moreover, PD patients with right-sided motor symptom onset frequently present with impairments in verbal memory and language, while patients with left-sided motor symptom onset frequently show impairments in visuospatial attention and mental imagery (Amick *et al.* 2006; Verreyt *et al.* 2011).

The relation of handedness and PD lesion onset side

One of the core findings linking PD to hemispheric asymmetries is an often-reported association between PD lesion onset side and handedness (Shi *et al.* 2014; Yust-Katz *et al.* 2008; Uitti *et al.* 2005). A systematic review and meta-analysis of this body of literature (van der Hoorn *et al.* 2012) revealed a clear association of handedness and PD lesion onset side. Overall, ten PD studies that involved data on handedness were identified, yielding an over-all sample size of 4405 PD patients. In this sample, 59.5% of right-handed patients showed right-dominant PD symptoms, while 40.5% showed left-dominant PD symptoms. This pattern was reversed for left-handed PD patients. In this group, 59.2% showed left-dominant PD symptoms, while 40.8% showed right-dominant PD symptoms. This relation was statistically significant with an odds ratio of 2.13, indicating that PD patients experience more symptoms on the side of their dominant hand. This suggests that the hemisphere dominant for fine motor coordination is more severely affected by PD than the non-dominant hemisphere. While the causal mechanisms underlying this intriguing observation remain a mystery, van der Hoorn *et al.* (2012) suggested that handedness could lead to increased metabolic demand in the contralateral hemisphere. This could result in increased oxidative stress and stronger dopaminergic defects in the dominant hemisphere. However, further research is needed to confirm this notion.

Psychophysiological paradigms

To date, only a few studies have used the dichotic listening paradigm in patients with PD. An early Norwegian study in 14 PD patients reported a reduced right ear advantage (REA) in PD patients compared to healthy controls (Hugdahl *et al.* 1990). Similar results were also found in a more recent longitudinal study on dichotic listening performance in PD patients (Sjöberg *et al.* 2015). Here, six PD patients who were treated with deep brain stimulation of the left subthalamic nucleus (STN) were tested with the dichotic listening task directly after surgery, and again at approximately 6- and 18-months post-surgery. The authors reported a decline of the REA over time, with three patients showing a REA before their surgeries and switching to a left ear advantage 18 months after surgery. Since both studies had very small sample sizes, more research on dichotic listening performance in PD is needed. Other psychophysiological laterality paradigms should be applied in PD for further insights into the disorder.

Functional hemispheric asymmetries in electrophysiological activity

One early study investigated hemispheric asymmetry in electroencephalogram (EEG) oscillations during sleep in seven PD patients but did not detect any significant hemispheric asymmetries (Myslobodsky *et al.* 1982). A more recent study investigated EEG oscillation asymmetries in 20 PD patients and 30 healthy controls during emotion processing (Yuvaraj *et al.* 2014). While emotion recognition was unimpaired in PD patients, they showed significant alterations in EEG alpha power asymmetries compared to controls. In general, both PD patients and controls showed rightward asymmetries in theta, alpha, and beta power. However, alpha power asymmetry was significantly reduced in PD patients for all brain regions compared to controls. A subsequent study in 34 PD patients and 18 healthy controls also reported reduced alpha power asymmetry in PD patients but only in the occipital lobe (Mostile *et al.* 2015). Interestingly, the extent of EEG alpha asymmetry correlated significantly with responsiveness to L-DOPA treatment. Here, a positive correlation was found indicating that PD patients with more pronounced alpha asymmetry were more responsive to treatment. The study also reported that relative to healthy controls PD patients showed stronger beta band asymmetries in frontal regions and also lower theta band asymmetries in frontal regions. Interestingly, there was a significant positive correlation between beta asymmetry and Hoehn-Yahr staging, a commonly used system to evaluate PD disease progress (Hoehn and Yahr 1967). Moreover, there was a significant negative correlation between theta asymmetry and Hoehn-Yahr staging. These findings suggest that frontal beta and theta asymmetries are associated with the extent of clinical disability in PD.

Functional hemispheric asymmetries in brain activation

Different neuroimaging techniques have been used to investigate hemispheric asymmetries in PD patients. For example, a recent study tested PD patients with an emotional prosody recognition task and assessed brain activity using a resting-state F-18 fluorodeoxyglucose positron emission tomography (PET) scan (Stirnimann *et al.* 2018). The authors found that patients with left-sided motor symptoms showed poorer vocal emotion recognition. At the metabolic level, they found that in patients with left-sided motor symptoms, there was a significant positive correlation between the metabolism of the right orbitofrontal cortex and happiness recognition. This shows that motor symptom asymmetry is an important predictor for emotion recognition in PD.

One study compared PD patients with left and right motor symptom onset using a feedback-based associative learning task and functional magnetic resonance imaging (fMRI) resting state (Huang *et al.* 2017). PD patients with right-sided onset of motor symptoms did not differ significantly from healthy controls. However, PD patients with a left-sided onset of motor symptoms made more acquisition errors in the task. Importantly, these errors showed an inverse relation with regional homogeneity in the right dorsal rostral putamen as assessed using resting state fMRI. This indicates that PD patients with a left-sided onset of motor symptoms may show a specific dysfunction of the right dorsal putamen that affects associative learning.

Interestingly, one fMRI study also showed an asymmetrical effect of L-DOPA medication on motor-related brain activity in PD patients (Martinu *et al.* 2014). In this study, right-handed PD patients performed finger movements with both their left and their right hands in the MRI scanner. In one condition they were tested while on L-DOPA medication, and in the other after a minimum of 12-hour medication withdrawal. Results showed that levodopa medication led to larger changes in neuronal activity for the non-dominant left hand. Here, significant activity differences after L-DOPA administration were observed in the motor cortico-striatal network which were not observed for right finger movements. These results show that it is important to include information on hemispheric asymmetries when assessing the effects of L-DOPA medication on PD symptoms.

Structural hemispheric asymmetries

To date, only few studies have investigated the relation between PD and altered structural hemispheric asymmetries in grey or white matter outside of the aforementioned asymmetry of substantia nigra neuronal loss (Kempster *et al.* 1989; Zhong *et al.* 2019). Interestingly, one study found a relation between side of PD motor symptom onset and lateralized grey matter volume loss in brain areas outside the substantia nigra (Lee *et al.* 2015). Using voxel-based morphometry, the authors found that patients with a left-sided onset of motor symptoms experienced grey matter loss predominantly in the precuneus and the superior occipital cortex of the right hemisphere.

However, a recent meta-analysis of grey matter asymmetries in aging and neurodegeneration did not report any consistent pattern of altered grey matter asymmetries in PD (Minkova *et al.* 2017). Regarding white matter, a recent analysis found that PD patients with left-sided onset of motor symptoms did not show any differences in white matter integrity compared to controls (Pelizzari *et al.* 2020). PD patients with right-sided onset of motor symptoms, however, showed widespread changes of white matter integrity, potentially leading to a less favourable prognosis.

Comparative research

Hemispheric asymmetries have been investigated in numerous studies involving animal models for PD, mostly in rodents. For example, it has been shown that mice with unilateral lesions of dopamine neurons in the medial forebrain bundle developed an asymmetry in grooming behaviour, with a reduction of grooming behaviour on the side contralateral to the lesion (Pelosi *et al.* 2015). These findings mirror the finding that human PD patients show motor impairments contralateral to lesions of dopaminergic neurons in the substantia nigra (Kempster *et al.* 1989). Similar results were also reported for other forms of hemispheric asymmetries, for example, forelimb placement asymmetries in rats (Landers *et al.* 2013, 2014). Interestingly, transplantation of induced pluripotent stem cells that had been differentiated into dopaminergic neurons into the rodent striatum led to a reduction of these behavioural asymmetries (Hargus *et al.* 2010). Taken together, comparative studies complement literature in human PD patients by further supporting the link between lesions in dopaminergic cells and motor symptom asymmetries.

Multiple sclerosis

Definition of the disorder

Multiple sclerosis (MS) is defined as an inflammatory demyelinating disease of the brain and spinal cord (Compston and Coles 2008). Characterized by damage to the myelin sheath (an insulation layer around axons), MS leads to neurological dysfunctions including physical and mental problems (Compston and Coles 2008). Multiple sclerosis is divided into four subtypes: clinically isolated syndrome, relapsing-remitting MS, primary progressive MS, and secondary progressive MS (Lublin *et al.* 2014). Symptoms are rated with the Expanded Disability Status Scale to characterise deficits in visual, brainstem, pyramidal, cerebellar, sensory, cerebral, and bowel/bladder functions as well as in movement (Kurtzke 1983). Symptoms include loss of cognitive and motor functions, visual and sensory problems as well as emotional problems leading to affective disorders, such as depression (Kurtzke 1983; Compston and Coles 2008).

MS is the most common inflammatory neurological disease in young adults with approximately 2.2 million people affected worldwide (Wallin *et al.* 2019). Interestingly, it is most common in people living farther from the equator and thus more frequent in northern European populations (Compston and Coles 2008). MS is a progressive, incurable disorder, and patients have a life expectancy of about 30 years upon onset. The female-to-male ratio is estimated to be roughly 2:1 (Wallin *et al.* 2019). Various genetic and environmental risk factors for MS have been discovered (Reich *et al.* 2018). High genetic risk in first-degree relatives (2–4%) and monozygotic twins (30–50%) has been found as well as multiple risk variants, with the human leukocyte antigen (HLA) *DRB1*1501* being the most prominent risk haplotype (Reich, Lucchinetti, and Calabresi 2018). Environmental risks include vitamin D deficits, tobacco exposure, and obesity (Reich *et al.* 2018). Several categories of drugs are used for the treatment of MS. Most act as immune-stimulating and antiviral and are most effective in the acute phases of MS (Reich *et al.* 2018). As MS is a neurological disorder that consequently deals with a progressive loss of function in different brain regions, MS allows investigation of neurodegenerative consequences on lateralization patterns.

Lesion laterality

While the effects of lesion laterality are a major topic in PD research, not much research on lesion laterality has been conducted in MS patients. One five-year longitudinal study in 66 MS patients and 16 healthy controls reported that, compared to patients who remained stable over the 5 years, patients who exhibited a worsening of clinical symptoms or cognitive decline showed a distinctly left-lateralized pattern of atrophies in both grey and white matter (Preziosa *et al.* 2017). Affected brain regions included deep grey matter, cortical regions in the frontal, temporal, parietal, and occipital lobes, the cerebellum, and several white matter tracts. The authors suggested that differential vulnerabilities of the two hemispheres to MS-related brain damage might affect clinical and cognitive worsening in MS, an intriguing finding that certainly deserves more empirical exploration.

Handedness

Left-handedness has been suggested to lead to increased risk of autoimmune and immune disorders (Geschwind and Behan 1982; Geschwind and Galaburda 1985a, 1985b, 1985c; Marx 1982)—a somewhat debated claim (Bryden *et al.* 1994; St-Marseille and Braun 1994). Since MS is an immune-mediated disease (Wootla *et al.* 2012), left-handedness has also been discussed as a potential risk factor for MS. For example, in a large study based on data from a prospective cohort study of 121,701 female nurses, 210 had confirmed cases of MS (Gardener *et al.* 2009). Comparing left-handers and right-handers from the overall cohort, left-handed women were found to have a 62% increased risk to be diagnosed with MS compared to right-handed women, a moderate but significant increase in MS risk. In contrast, a recent study that directly assessed left-handedness in a cohort of 8888 MS patients did find a rate of left-handedness of 10.3% in MS patients (Shirani *et al.* 2019), which is very close to what is observed in the general population. The authors concluded that there are no prognostic implications of left-handedness for MS. More research in even larger cohorts is needed to draw a final conclusion on this matter.

Psychophysiological paradigms

Several studies have used the dichotic listening paradigm in patients with MS and results seem to be consistent. For example, an early study from the 1980s found a reduction of left-ear answers, for example, a stronger REA in 11 right-handed MS patients compared to right-handed controls (Rubens *et al.* 1985; Musiek *et al.* 1989). Similar results were also obtained in other studies (Lindeboom and ter Horst 1988; Musiek *et al.* 1989; Wishart *et al.* 1995). Only one study reported a left ear advantage (LEA) in individuals with MS in a dichotic digits test (Peñaloza López *et al.* 2018). Several MRI studies subsequently found that only those MS patients who actually showed atrophy of the corpus callosum (CC) had left ear suppression (Rao *et al.* 1989; Pelletier *et al.* 1993; Barkhof *et al.* 1998; Gadea *et al.* 2002). This may explain why one of the mentioned behavioural studies did not find a stronger REA in MS patients. One longitudinal MRI study reported a significant progressive loss of posterior CC areas (isthmus and splenium) over time that was related to a stronger REA over time (Gadea *et al.* 2009). Taken together, the literature suggests that MS-related disconnection or atrophy of auditory pathways in the CC leads to a stronger REA in dichotic listening. This may be caused by the fact that information from the left ear is initially processed by the right hemisphere and, in most individuals, needs to be transferred over the CC to the language-dominant left hemisphere. If this transfer is impaired, the REA increases.

Structural hemispheric asymmetries

Only very few studies have investigated structural asymmetries in grey matter in MS. One voxel-based morphometry study in 51 patients with relapsing-remitting MS and 34 healthy controls found that, compared to controls, MS patients showed grey matter reductions in left fronto-temporal structures and in deep grey matter (Prinster *et al.* 2006). Another, more recent study used diffusion tensor imaging (DTI) to compare fractional anisotropy, a commonly used diffusion parameter, in four brain areas (Cerebral peduncle, thalamus, caudate nucleus, centrum semiovale) between MS patients with primary progressive MS and relapsing-remitting MS (Savio *et al.* 2015). Here, patients with relapsing-remitting MS showed significant asymmetries in the thalamus and caudate nucleus, but the implications of this finding remain rather unclear.

Comparative research

We could only identify a single comparative study that was focused on laterality in an animal model for MS (Tambalo *et al.* 2015). The authors used fMRI in rats with experimental autoimmune encephalomyelitis (EAE), a preclinical model of chronic MS. They found that during somatosensory stimulation of the right forepaw, the rats showed reduced lateralization of brain activation in motor areas compared to baseline.

Alzheimer's disease

Definition of the disorder

First described in 1906 by the physician Alois Alzheimer, AD is the most common neurodegenerative disorder worldwide and affects about 6% of people aged 65 years and older (Wallin *et al.* 2019; Burns and Iliffe 2009). It is defined by a progressive decline of memory and cognitive abilities (WHO 2016). More precisely, AD is characterized by three main symptom categories. These include cognitive dysfunction, such as memory loss and language problems, and psychiatric symptoms, such as depression, hallucinations, or delusions. The third group of symptoms is difficulty when performing daily activities, such as dressing, eating, and shopping (Burns and Iliffe 2009). Alzheimer's disease is the most common cause of dementia (Burns and Iliffe 2009), and the global disability caused by dementia is higher than for almost any other disease (Alzheimer's Association 2019; Ferri *et al.* 2005). The cause of AD is primarily the loss of neurons and synapses in the cerebral cortex and subcortical regions leading to atrophy (Ballard *et al.* 2011). Alzheimer's disease is a protein misfolding disease, and two core pathological alterations discussed as responsible for this loss of neurons are the accumulation of amyloid plaques and neurofibrillary tangles (Ballard *et al.* 2011). Amyloid plaques result from amyloid-beta (Aβ) protein which is part of the amyloid precursor protein (APP). In AD, APP is falsely disassembled, and resulting Aβ proteins accumulate and form neurotoxic plaques. Aggregation of the tau protein leads to neurofibrillary tangles inside the cell body destroying the cytoskeleton of the cell (Ballard *et al.* 2011). Early-onset AD (onset < 65 years) is most likely caused by mutations in the *APP*, *PSEN1*, or *PSEN2* genes and is highly heritable (mostly autosomal dominantly inherited). Mutations in these genes lead most certainly to Aβ aggregation and thus AD (Reitz and Mayeux 2014). Overall, most AD cases are late-onset AD (onset > 65 years), which still holds a two-fold increased risk when a first-degree relative has AD (Reitz and Mayeux 2014). Moreover, several risk genes for developing AD have been identified, including *APOE, GSK3β, Tau,* and *DYRK1A* (Ballard *et al.* 2011). These are all involved in creating or accumulating either amyloid plaques or neurofibrillary tangles. Environmental risk factors for AD include previous cerebrovascular diseases, type 2 diabetes, and smoking (Reitz and Mayeux 2014). The disorder is divided into three stages. First, the preclinical AD, then mild cognitive impairment due to AD, and finally dementia due to AD (Alzheimer's Association 2019). Treatment mainly targets cognitive symptoms; thus cholinesterase inhibitors and NMDA receptor antagonists are frequently prescribed, but drugs targeting the protein misfolding process are being tested (Ballard *et al.* 2011).

Asymmetries of amyloid-β burden

Regarding laterality and AD, it is of interest that neuronal atrophy frequently has an asymmetrical beginning and that side of atrophy onset might predict symptom severity. For example, one study investigated lateralized Aβ burden and its relation to lateralized neurodegeneration and cognitive impairment (Frings *et al.* 2015). The authors found that hypometabolism was more pronounced on the side of greater Aβ burden in 6 out of 25 investigated brain regions (angular gyrus, middle frontal gyrus, middle occipital gyrus, superior parietal gyrus, inferior and middle temporal gyrus). Asymmetry of Aβ burden was also related to cognitive impairments, with a stronger leftward asymmetry of Aβ burden related to more severe language impairment. In contrast, stronger rightward asymmetry of Aβ deposition was associated with more severe visuospatial impairment. These findings show that asymmetries of Aβ burden in AD are associated with impairments in lateralized cognitive systems such as language and visuospatial processing.

Handedness

Several studies have investigated the association between handedness and AD. For example, one early study in 65 men with AD reported a significantly higher prevalence of left-handedness in patients with early-onset AD but not in patients with late-onset AD (Seltzer *et al.* 1984). In contrast, a subsequent study in 114 AD patients and 217 healthy controls found a reduced frequency of left-handedness in AD (only 2.6%) compared to healthy controls (11.1%) (De Leon *et al.* 1986). A Chinese study in 70 AD patients and 140 healthy controls did not find any relation between AD and handedness (Li *et al.* 1992), while a Finnish twin study reported a non-significant trend towards an association between ambidexterity or left-handedness and AD (Räihä *et al.* 1998). One study that looked into specific symptoms of AD in

18 left-handed and 18 right-handed AD patients found that the severity or pattern of neuropsychological deficits did not differ between the two groups, but that left-handedness might contribute to early AD onset (Doody *et al*. 1999). The largest and most recent study on handedness in AD assessed a cohort of 182 AD patients and 256 healthy controls and did not find any difference between handedness frequencies in AD patients and healthy controls (Ryan *et al*. 2020). Altogether, the existing evidence suggests that it is unlikely that there is a strong association between left-handedness and AD, but more research in larger cohorts is needed before any final conclusions can be drawn.

Psychophysiological paradigms

Functional hemispheric asymmetries in AD patients have been investigated using the dichotic listening paradigm. One study found that AD patients showed a larger REA than healthy controls (Duchek and Balota 2005). The authors suggested that this finding may indicate a tendency to respond to the stimulus initially processed by the speech-dominant left hemisphere in AD patients. This finding may be related to a decrease in interhemispheric transfer due to atrophy of the CC. Most studies, however, find that the main difference between AD patients and healthy controls in dichotic listening performance lies in attention allocation. A review article on dichotic listening in AD (Bouma and Gootjes 2011) synthesised the relevant literature and found that AD patients showed a severe deficit in allocating attention to the left ear (e.g. in processing speech information with the non-language-dominant right hemisphere). This results in an REA even in trials in which attention should be focused on the left ear. The authors concluded that both callosal atrophy and subcortical lesions within the hemispheres contribute to this issue.

Functional hemispheric asymmetries in brain activation

Using PET, Duara *et al*. (1986) found a significant increase in right-to-left metabolic asymmetry in AD patients compared to controls, particularly in the parietal lobe. A more recent study with resting state fMRI found that AD patients showed average rightward lateralization during resting state fMRI, while healthy controls showed leftward lateralization (Liu *et al*. 2018). This rightward shift in resting-state asymmetry might be related to compensation mechanisms for AD-related brain damage in the left hemisphere. A dichotic listening study in the MR scanner found that AD patients showed an increased REA and decreased callosal size compared to healthy controls (Gootjes *et al*. 2006). Importantly, controls showed a significant correlation between dichotic listening performance and CC size that was absent in AD patients. This suggests that callosal atrophy is not the only mechanism that affects the changes in the REA observed in AD patients.

Structural hemispheric asymmetries

A substantial number of studies have investigated structural hemispheric asymmetries in AD. A recent meta-analysis of voxel-based morphometry studies on grey matter asymmetries in aging and neurodegeneration included 63 experiments in AD patients groups with an overall N of 1430 (Minkova *et al.* 2017). Here, the authors found evidence for a bilateral loss of grey matter in the hippocampus that was more pronounced in the left hemisphere. Additionally, the superior and middle temporal gyri showed atrophies that were more pronounced in the right hemisphere. A more recent neurogenetic study in 1241 AD patients (Wachinger *et al.* 2018) reported AD-related increases in shape asymmetry in the hippocampus, amygdala, and putamen. These asymmetry increases were associated with genetic variation of single nucleotide polymorphisms in several genes that had previously been associated with either AD diagnosis or brain subcortical volume, indicating a molecular link between AD pathogenesis and hemispheric asymmetries. Moreover, another neuroimaging study linked the AD-related gene *APOE* to hemispheric asymmetries (Donix *et al.* 2013). In this study, *APOE*-4 allele carriers (a risk variant for AD) were found to have a thinner left than right entorhinal cortex compared to other genotypes.

Structural hemispheric asymmetries in AD have been linked to symptom severity. For example, one study reported that specifically, atrophy of the left ventral thalamus was relevant for disease severity in AD (Low *et al.* 2019b). Another study by the same group reported greater leftward occipital white matter asymmetries in AD patients compared to controls, which was also associated with poorer performance in tests of cognition, memory, language, and executive functions (Low *et al.* 2019a). Moreover, a link between hippocampal asymmetry and dementia severity has been reported (Ardekani *et al.* 2019).

Comparative models

So far, hemispheric asymmetries have not been a major focus of comparative AD studies. One recent study investigated asymmetries of fibrillar plaque burden in five different amyloid mouse models (Sacher *et al.* 2020). Here, the authors found that more than 30% of investigated models showed substantial asymmetries in fibrillar plaque burden. This finding complements the previously described findings in humans in showing that asymmetric disease burden is a common phenomenon in AD.

Conclusion

Taken together, empirical evidence suggests that laterality of lesion onset in PD (and to a lesser extent in MS) is a variable that should always be considered in the clinical assessment of these degenerative disorders and neuroscientific research on their causes and consequences. Similarly, asymmetries are a relevant factor in AD. Regarding functional hemispheric asymmetries, the main finding in neurological disorders is the high relevance of handedness in PD. Moreover, unlike what has been described in neurodevelopmental and psychiatric disorders, neurological disorders are not typically associated with reduced hemispheric asymmetries but can result in enhanced hemispheric asymmetries as in the case of language lateralization in AD. This may be due to structural atrophy enhancing unihemispheric processing, resulting in stronger functional hemispheric asymmetries.

References

Agosta, S., *et al.*, 2020. Lateralized cognitive functions in Parkinson's patients: a behavioral approach for the early detection of sustained attention deficits. *Brain Research*, 1726, 146486.

Alzheimer's Association, 2019. 2019 Alzheimer's disease facts and figures. *Alzheimer's & Dementia*, 15 (3), 321–387.

Amick, M.M., Grace, J., and Chou, K.L., 2006. Body side of motor symptom onset in Parkinson's disease is associated with memory performance. *Journal of the International Neuropsychological Society: JINS*, 12 (5), 736–740.

Ardekani, B.A., *et al.*, 2019. Sexual dimorphism and hemispheric asymmetry of hippocampal volumetric integrity in normal aging and Alzheimer disease. *AJNR. American Journal of Neuroradiology*, 40 (2), 276–282.

Ballard, C., *et al.*, 2011. Alzheimer's disease. *The Lancet*, 377 (9770), 1019–1031.

Barkhof, F.J., *et al.*, 1998. Functional correlates of callosal atrophy in relapsing-remitting multiple sclerosis patients. A preliminary MRI study. *Journal of Neurology*, 245 (3), 153–158.

Bellou, V., *et al.*, 2016. Environmental risk factors and Parkinson's disease: an umbrella review of meta-analyses. *Parkinsonism & Related Disorders*, 23, 1–9.

Blauwendraat, C., Nalls, M.A., and Singleton, A.B., 2020. The genetic architecture of Parkinson's disease. *The Lancet Neurology*, 19 (2), 170–178.

Bouma, A., and Gootjes, L., 2011. Effects of attention on dichotic listening in elderly and patients with dementia of the Alzheimer type. *Brain and Cognition*, 76 (2), 286–293.

Bryden, M.P., McManus, I.C., and Bulman-Fleming, M.B., 1994. Evaluating the empirical support for the Geschwind-Behan-Galaburda model of cerebral lateralization. *Brain and Cognition*, 26 (2), 103–167.

Burns, A., and Iliffe, S., 2009. Alzheimer's disease. *BMJ (Clinical Research Ed.)*, 338, b158.

Compston, A., and Coles, A., 2008. Multiple sclerosis. *The Lancet*, 372 (9648), 1502–1517.

Cronin-Golomb, A., 2010. Parkinson's disease as a disconnection syndrome. *Neuropsychology Review*, 20 (2), 191–208.

De Leon, M.J., *et al.*, 1986. Reduced incidence of left-handedness in clinically diagnosed dementia of the Alzheimer type. *Neurobiology of Aging*, 7 (3), 161–164.

De Rijk, M.C., *et al.*, 2000. Prevalence of Parkinson's disease in Europe: a collaborative study of population-based cohorts. Neurologic Diseases in the Elderly Research Group. *Neurology*, 54 (11 Suppl 5), S21–S23.

Djaldetti, R., Ziv, I., and Melamed, E., 2006. The mystery of motor asymmetry in Parkinson's disease. *The Lancet. Neurology*, 5 (9), 796–802.

Donix, M., *et al.*, 2013. APOE associated hemispheric asymmetry of entorhinal cortical thickness in aging and Alzheimer's disease. *Psychiatry Research*, 214 (3), 212–220.

Doody, R.S., *et al.*, 1999. The influence of handedness on the clinical presentation and neuropsychology of Alzheimer disease. *Archives of Neurology*, 56 (9), 1133–1137.

Duara, R., *et al.*, 1986. Positron emission tomography in Alzheimer's disease. *Neurology*, 36 (7), 879–887.

Duchek, J.M., and Balota, D.A., 2005. Failure to control prepotent pathways in early stage dementia of the Alzheimer's type: evidence from dichotic listening. *Neuropsychology*, 19 (5), 687–695.

Ferri, C.P., *et al.*, 2005. Global prevalence of dementia: a Delphi consensus study. *Lancet*, 366 (9503), 2112–2117.

Frings, L., *et al.*, 2015. Asymmetries of amyloid-β burden and neuronal dysfunction are positively correlated in Alzheimer's disease. *Brain: A Journal of Neurology*, 138 (Pt 10), 3089–3099.

Gadea, M., *et al.*, 2002. Dichotic listening and corpus callosum magnetic resonance imaging in relapsing-remitting multiple sclerosis with emphasis on sex differences. *Neuropsychology*, 16 (2), 275–281.

Gadea, M., *et al.*, 2009. Corpus callosum function in verbal dichotic listening: inferences from a longitudinal follow-up of Relapsing-Remitting Multiple Sclerosis patients. *Brain and Language*, 110 (2), 101–105.

Gardener, H., *et al.*, 2009. The relationship between handedness and risk of multiple sclerosis. *Multiple Sclerosis (Houndmills, Basingstoke, England)*, 15 (5), 587–592.

Geschwind, N., and Behan, P., 1982. Left-handedness: association with immune disease, migraine, and developmental learning disorder. *Proceedings of the National Academy of Sciences of the United States of America*, 79 (16), 5097–5100.

Geschwind, N., and Galaburda, A.M., 1985a. Cerebral lateralization. Biological mechanisms, associations, and pathology: I. A hypothesis and a program for research. *Archives of Neurology*, 42 (5), 428–459.

Geschwind, N., and Galaburda, A.M., 1985b. Cerebral lateralization. Biological mechanisms, associations, and pathology: II. A hypothesis and a program for research. *Archives of Neurology*, 42 (6), 521–552.

Geschwind, N., and Galaburda, A.M., 1985c. Cerebral lateralization. Biological mechanisms, associations, and pathology: III. A hypothesis and a program for research. *Archives of Neurology*, 42 (7), 634–654.

Gómez-Esteban, J.C., *et al.*, 2010. Factors influencing the symmetry of Parkinson's disease symptoms. *Clinical Neurology and Neurosurgery*, 112 (4), 302–305.

Gootjes, L., *et al.*, 2006. Corpus callosum size correlates with asymmetric performance on a dichotic listening task in healthy aging but not in Alzheimer's disease. *Neuropsychologia*, 44 (2), 208–217.

Hargus, G., *et al.*, 2010. Differentiated Parkinson patient-derived induced pluripotent stem cells grow in the adult rodent brain and reduce motor asymmetry in Parkinsonian rats. *Proceedings of the National Academy of Sciences of the United States of America*, 107 (36), 15921–15926.

Hoehn, M.M., and Yahr, M.D., 1967. Parkinsonism: onset, progression and mortality. *Neurology*, 17 (5), 427–442.

Huang, P., *et al.*, 2017. Motor-symptom laterality affects acquisition in Parkinson's disease: a cognitive and functional magnetic resonance imaging study. *Movement Disorders: Official Journal of the Movement Disorder Society*, 32 (7), 1047–1055.

Hugdahl, K., Wester, K., and Asbjørnsen, A., 1990. The role of the left and right thalamus in language asymmetry: dichotic listening in Parkinson patients undergoing stereotactic thalamotomy. *Brain and Language*, 39 (1), 1–13.

Kalia, L.V., and Lang, A.E., 2015. Parkinson's disease. *The Lancet*, 386 (9996), 896–912.

Kempster, P.A., *et al.*, 1989. Asymmetry of substantia nigra neuronal loss in Parkinson's disease and its relevance to the mechanism of levodopa related motor fluctuations. *Journal of Neurology, Neurosurgery, and Psychiatry*, 52 (1), 72–76.

Kurtzke, J.F., 1983. Rating neurologic impairment in multiple sclerosis. *Neurology*, 33 (11), 1444.

Landers, M.R., *et al.*, 2013. A comparison of voluntary and forced exercise in protecting against behavioral asymmetry in a juvenile hemi Parkinsonian rat model. *Behavioural Brain Research*, 248, 121–128.

Landers, M.R., Kinney, J.W., and van Breukelen, F., 2014. Forced exercise before or after induction of 6-OHDA-mediated nigrostriatal insult does not mitigate behavioral asymmetry in a hemi Parkinsonian rat model. *Brain Research*, 1543, 263–270.

Lee, E.-Y., *et al.*, 2015. Side of motor onset is associated with hemisphere-specific memory decline and lateralized gray matter loss in Parkinson's disease. *Parkinsonism & Related Disorders*, 21 (5), 465–470.

Li, G., *et al.*, 1992. A case-control study of Alzheimer's disease in China. *Neurology*, 42 (8), 1481–1488.

Lindeboom, J., and ter Horst, R., 1988. Interhemispheric disconnection effects in multiple sclerosis. *Journal of Neurology, Neurosurgery, and Psychiatry*, 51 (11), 1445–1447.

Liu, H., *et al.*, 2018. Changes in brain lateralization in patients with mild cognitive impairment and Alzheimer's disease: a resting-state functional magnetic resonance study from Alzheimer's disease neuroimaging initiative. *Frontiers in Neurology*, 9, 3.

Low, A., *et al.*, 2019a. Association of asymmetrical white matter hyperintensities and apolipoprotein E4 on cognitive impairment. *Journal of Alzheimer's Disease: JAD*, 70 (3), 953–964.

Low, A., *et al.*, 2019b. Asymmetrical atrophy of thalamic subnuclei in Alzheimer's disease and amyloid-positive mild cognitive impairment is associated with key clinical features. *Alzheimer's & Dementia (Amsterdam, Netherlands)*, 11, 690–699.

Lublin, F.D., *et al.*, 2014. Defining the clinical course of multiple sclerosis: the 2013 revisions. *Neurology*, 83 (3), 278–286.

Martinu, K., *et al.*, 2014. Asymmetrical effect of levodopa on the neural activity of motor regions in PD. *PLoS One*, 9 (11), e111600.

Marx, J.L., 1982. Autoimmunity in left-handers. Left-handedness may be associated with an increased risk of autoimmune disease. Is testosterone the link between the two? *Science (New York, N.Y.)*, 217 (4555), 141–142, 144.

Minkova, L., *et al.*, 2017. Gray matter asymmetries in aging and neurodegeneration: a review and meta-analysis. *Human Brain Mapping*, 38 (12), 5890–5904.

Mostile, G., *et al.*, 2015. Electroencephalographic lateralization, clinical correlates and pharmacological response in untreated Parkinson's disease. *Parkinsonism & Related Disorders*, 21 (8), 948–953.

Musiek, F.E., *et al.*, 1989. Electrophysiologic and behavioral auditory findings in multiple sclerosis. *The American Journal of Otology*, 10 (5), 343–350.

Myslobodsky, M., *et al.*, 1982. Unilateral dopamine deficit and lateral EEG asymmetry: sleep abnormalities in hemi-Parkinson's patients. *Electroencephalography and Clinical Neurophysiology*, 54 (2), 227–231.

Pelizzari, L., *et al.*, 2020. White matter alterations in early Parkinson's disease: role of motor symptom lateralization. *Neurological Sciences: Official Journal of the Italian Neurological Society and of the Italian Society of Clinical Neurophysiology*, 41 (2), 357–364.

Pelletier, J., *et al.*, 1993. Functional and magnetic resonance imaging correlates of callosal involvement in multiple sclerosis. *Archives of Neurology*, 50 (10), 1077–1082.

Pelosi, A., Girault, J.-A., and Hervé, D., 2015. Unilateral lesion of dopamine neurons induces grooming asymmetry in the mouse. *PLoS One*, 10 (9), e0137185.

Peñaloza López, Y.R., Orozco Peña, X.D., and Pérez Ruiz, S.J., 2018. Esclerosis múltiple: ventaja izquierda para la lateralidad auditiva en pruebas dicóticas de procesamiento auditivo central y relación de pruebas psicoacústicas con examen de discapacidad-EDEM. *Acta otorrinolaringologica espanola*, 69 (6), 325–330.

Poewe, W., 2008. Non-motor symptoms in Parkinson's disease. *European Journal of Neurology*, 15 (Suppl 1), 14–20.

Preziosa, P., *et al.*, 2017. Progression of regional atrophy in the left hemisphere contributes to clinical and cognitive deterioration in multiple sclerosis: a 5-year study. *Human Brain Mapping*, 38 (11), 5648–5665.

Prinster, A., *et al.*, 2006. Grey matter loss in relapsing-remitting multiple sclerosis: a voxel-based morphometry study. *NeuroImage*, 29 (3), 859–867.

Räihä, I., *et al.*, 1998. Environmental differences in twin pairs discordant for Alzheimer's disease. *Journal of Neurology, Neurosurgery, and Psychiatry*, 65 (5), 785–787.

Rao, S.M., *et al.*, 1989. Cerebral disconnection in multiple sclerosis. Relationship to atrophy of the corpus callosum. *Archives of Neurology*, 46 (8), 918–920.

Reich, D.S., Lucchinetti, C.F., and Calabresi, P.A., 2018. Multiple sclerosis. *The New England Journal of Medicine*, 378 (2), 169–180.

Reitz, C., and Mayeux, R., 2014. Alzheimer disease: epidemiology, diagnostic criteria, risk factors and biomarkers. *Biochemical Pharmacology*, 88 (4), 640–651.

Riederer, P., *et al.*, 2018. Lateralisation in Parkinson disease. *Cell and Tissue Research*, 373 (1), 297–312.

Riederer, P., and Sian-Hülsmann, J., 2012. The significance of neuronal lateralisation in Parkinson's disease. *Journal of Neural Transmission (Vienna, Austria: 1996)*, 119 (8), 953–962.

Rubens, A.B., *et al.*, 1985. Left ear suppression on verbal dichotic tests in patients with multiple sclerosis. *Annals of Neurology*, 18 (4), 459–463.

Ryan, J.J., Kreiner, D.S., and Paolo, A.M., 2020. Handedness of healthy elderly and patients with Alzheimer's disease. *The International Journal of Neuroscience*, 1–9.

Sacher, C., *et al.*, 2020. Asymmetry of fibrillar plaque burden in amyloid mouse models. *Journal of Nuclear Medicine: Official Publication, Society of Nuclear Medicine*, 61, 1825–1831.

Savio, S., *et al.*, 2015. Hemispheric asymmetry measured by texture analysis and diffusion tensor imaging in two multiple sclerosis subtypes. *Acta Radiologica (Stockholm, Sweden: 1987)*, 56 (7), 844–851.

Seltzer, B., Burres, M.J., and Sherwin, I., 1984. Left-handedness in early and late onset dementia. *Neurology*, 34 (3), 367–369.

Shi, J., Liu, J., and Qu, Q., 2014. Handedness and dominant side of symptoms in Parkinson's disease. *Medicina Clinica*, 142 (4), 141–144.

Shirani, A., Cross, A.H., and Naismith, R.T., 2019. The association between handedness and clinicodemographic characteristics in people with multiple sclerosis: a brief report. *Multiple Sclerosis Journal—Experimental, Translational and Clinical*, 5 (1), 2055217319832031.

Sjöberg, R.L., *et al.*, 2015. Laterality and deep brain stimulation of the subthalamic nucleus: applying a dichotic listening task to patients treated for Parkinson's disease. *Neurocase*, 21 (5), 601–606.

Stirnimann, N., *et al.*, 2018. Hemispheric specialization of the basal ganglia during vocal emotion decoding: evidence from asymmetric Parkinson's disease and 18FDG PET. *Neuropsychologia*, 119, 1–11.

St-Marseille, A., and Braun, C.M., 1994. Comments on immune aspects of the Geschwind-Behan-Galaburda model and of the article of Bryden, McManus, and Bulman-Fleming. *Brain and Cognition*, 26 (2), 281–290.

Sveinbjornsdottir, S., 2016. The clinical symptoms of Parkinson's disease. *Journal of Neurochemistry*, 139 (Suppl 1), 318–324.

Tambalo, S., *et al.*, 2015. Functional magnetic resonance imaging of rats with experimental autoimmune encephalomyelitis reveals brain cortex remodeling. *The Journal of Neuroscience: The Official Journal of the Society for Neuroscience*, 35 (27), 10088–10100.

Tysnes, O.-B., and Storstein, A., 2017. Epidemiology of Parkinson's disease. *Journal of Neural Transmission (Vienna, Austria: 1996)*, 124 (8), 901–905.

Uitti, R.J., *et al.*, 2005. Parkinson disease: handedness predicts asymmetry. *Neurology*, 64 (11), 1925–1930.

van der Hoorn, A., *et al.*, 2012. Handedness correlates with the dominant Parkinson side: a systematic review and meta-analysis. *Movement Disorders: Official Journal of the Movement Disorder Society*, 27 (2), 206–210.

Verreyt, N., *et al.*, 2011. Cognitive differences between patients with left-sided and right-sided Parkinson's disease. A review. *Neuropsychology Review*, 21 (4), 405–424.

Wachinger, C., *et al.*, 2018. A longitudinal imaging genetics study of neuroanatomical asymmetry in Alzheimer's disease. *Biological Psychiatry*, 84 (7), 522–530.

Wallin, M.T., *et al.*, 2019. Global, regional, and national burden of multiple sclerosis 1990–2016: a systematic analysis for the Global Burden of Disease Study 2016. *The Lancet. Neurology*, 18 (3), 269–285.

WHO, 2016. International classification of disease-10. Available from: https://icd.who.int/browse10/2016/en.

Wishart, H.A., *et al.*, 1995. Interhemispheric transfer in multiple sclerosis. *Journal of Clinical and Experimental Neuropsychology*, 17 (6), 937–940.

Wootla, B., Eriguchi, M., and Rodriguez, M., 2012. Is multiple sclerosis an autoimmune disease? *Autoimmune Diseases*, 2012, 969657.

Yust-Katz, S., *et al.*, 2008. Handedness as a predictor of side of onset of Parkinson's disease. *Parkinsonism & Related Disorders*, 14 (8), 633–635.

Yuvaraj, R., *et al.*, 2014. On the analysis of EEG power, frequency and asymmetry in Parkinson's disease during emotion processing. *Behavioral and Brain Functions: BBF*, 10, 12.

Zhong, Z., *et al.*, 2019. High-spatial-resolution diffusion MRI in Parkinson disease: lateral asymmetry of the substantia Nigra. *Radiology*, 291 (1), 149–157.

5 Integration and outlook

A transdiagnostic perspective on clinical laterality research

Introduction

Why do scientists investigate hemispheric asymmetries in clinical groups? Many studies explicitly mention or indirectly imply that clinical laterality research could benefit patients suffering from these disorders. This could happen on different levels. On the one hand, the results of clinical laterality research could directly benefit individual patients, for example by optimizing therapeutic interventions or enabling an earlier diagnosis. On the other hand, clinical laterality research could contribute to a better understanding of how these disorders emerge or can be treated from a basic science perspective. This would then benefit individual patients more indirectly. In this chapter, we will shortly discuss these different viewpoints and evaluate them in the context of the published literature discussed in the previous chapters.

Can clinical laterality research help improve therapeutic interventions?

The relevance of hemispheric asymmetries for therapeutic interventions for neurodevelopmental and psychiatric disorders has been suggested on two levels (Ocklenburg *et al.* 2020). First, it has been suggested that many psychotherapeutic interventions focus largely on "left-hemispheric functions" like logic language and that psychotherapy could benefit from integrating "right-hemispheric functions" like creativity to a larger extent (Banmen 1983). For example, this idea has been explained in detail in a recent book by Allan N. Schore (2019). While these ideas certainly are interesting, we are currently not aware of any clinical studies that empirically tested whether such approaches would indeed enhance therapy efficiency and patient well-being. Therefore, these ideas remain on the theoretical level, but it would certainly be interesting to see future empirical studies investigating them. Second, it has been suggested that individual differences in hemispheric asymmetries could influence therapy outcome. For example, it has been shown that mixed-handed Vietnam veterans suffering from post traumatic stress disorder (PTSD) benefited significantly less from psychosocial interventions than veterans that were clearly left- or right-handed (Forbes *et al.* 2006). Moreover, a study on depression found that depressed patients that responded to cognitive behavioural therapy showed a left-hemispheric dominance on a dichotic fused words test that was more than twice as large as in non-responders (Kishon *et al.* 2015). This suggests that strong left-hemispheric language dominance may be beneficial for therapy outcome. Interestingly, a similar relation has also been reported for the treatment of depression with the antidepressant fluoxetine (Bruder 1996; Bruder *et al.* 2004). Most recently, a study on alcoholism found that crossed hand and eye laterality, as well as left-eyedness, was related to a reduced risk for alcohol-related readmission in a sample of 200 early-abstinent alcohol-dependent inpatients (Weinland *et al.* 2019). Taken together, there clearly is a need for a larger amount of clinical laterality studies that directly assess the relevance of hemispheric asymmetries in the context of therapy. Existing studies provide many exciting leads, but more systematic research in larger cohorts is needed before any final conclusions can be drawn.

Can clinical laterality research help improve diagnostics for specific disorders?

In addition to the relevance of hemispheric asymmetries for therapeutic interventions, it has been suggested that consideration of asymmetries might be helpful in the context of diagnosing neurodevelopmental, psychiatric, and neurological disorders. The main idea in this context is that atypical hemispheric asymmetries may represent so-called biomarkers that could improve the identification of individuals who are at risk of developing a certain disorder in preclinical stages (Oertel-Knöchel *et al.* 2012). This identification at a preclinical stage would then allow for an earlier start of targeted interventions and, resulting from that, improved patient wellbeing. The most prominent example for such a biomarker hypothesis in clinical laterality research may be the idea that atypical functional and structural asymmetries may represent a biomarker for schizophrenia, as brought forward by Oertel-Knöchel *et al.* (2012).

The two main questions in whether or not atypical hemispheric asymmetries represent useful biomarkers for the emergence of neurodevelopmental, psychiatric, or neurological disorders relate to how specific the relation between laterality and pathology is. On the one hand, a useful biomarker for the development of neurodevelopmental, psychiatric, and neurological disorders should have a high chance of being present in individuals who develop such disorders but have a high chance of being absent in individuals who do not develop such disorders. Thus, it should not only be possible to predict who will develop a disorder but also who will not develop a disorder. On the other hand, a useful biomarker for a specific disorder should also not only differentiate between low-risk and high-risk individuals for developing any sort of psychopathology but also differentiate specific risk for one disorder against other disorders.

Importantly, however, atypical hemispheric asymmetries can not only be found in patients suffering from these disorders but also in healthy individuals. This can be exemplified using handedness. Recently, a large-scale meta-analysis reported that in the general population the rate of left-handedness was 10.6% while the rate of right-handedness was 89.4% when studies using a two-categories classification scheme were analysed (Papadatou-Pastou *et al.* 2020). When studies that used a three-categories classification scheme (left, right, mixed) were analysed, the percentage of non-right-handedness was 18.1% and the percentage of right-handedness was 81.9%. Compared to that, a recent meta-analysis of handedness in autism spectrum disorders (ASD) (Markou *et al.* 2017) revealed elevated levels of atypical handedness. In this meta-analysis, individuals with ASD showed a prevalence of non-right-handedness of 45.4%, more than double the prevalence in healthy individuals. However, as ASD affects only about 1% of the general population (see Chapter 2), the vast majority of people who are left-handed or mixed-handed will be healthy and not suffering from ASD. Thus, on its own, non-right-handedness is not a specific biomarker for ASD or any other neurodevelopmental, psychiatric, or neurological disorder.

Moreover, the literature reviewed in the preceding chapters revealed that with few exceptions, almost all forms of hemispheric asymmetries that showed robust empirical evidence (e.g. significant effects on the meta-analytic level or in several high-powered individual studies) for being altered in any neurodevelopmental, psychiatric, or neurological disorder showed an increase of atypical asymmetries. For example, a higher rate of non-right-handedness has not only been reported in ASD but also in several other disorders including schizophrenia (see Chapter 3). Thus, altered hemispheric asymmetries do not represent a biomarker that is specific for any disorder. The fact that alterations in the same direction (higher prevalence of atypical hemispheric asymmetries) have been observed in many different disorders presents an interesting finding in the context of transdiagnostic approaches. Moreover, it hints at a relationship between atypical hemispheric asymmetries and a general risk to develop psychopathology outside of specific diagnosis. However, also for this relationship, the fact that most individuals who show atypical hemispheric asymmetries are healthy represents a major obstacle for any use as a biomarker or predictor.

Are atypical hemispheric asymmetries cause, consequence, or correlate of neurodevelopmental, psychiatric, and neurological disorders?

The empirical evidence presented in the previous chapters clearly indicates that there is a statistical association between atypical hemispheric asymmetries and many different neurodevelopmental, psychiatric, and neurological disorders. This leaves the question of whether there is a causal relation between hemispheric asymmetries and disorders. For handedness, an influential early model for the relation of pathology and hemispheric asymmetries proposed by Paul Satz suggested that early brain damage could lead to a switch in handedness (Satz 1972). This would lead to a higher probability of left-handedness having a pathological cause due to the higher prevalence of right-handedness in the population. To what extent this model is applicable in the context of neurodevelopmental and psychiatric disorders is, however, largely unclear, as most patients suffering from these disorders do not show overt brain damage.

For neurodevelopmental and psychiatric disorders, Dorothy Bishop identified four possible causal or non-causal relationships between atypical hemispheric asymmetries and diagnosis of a disorder using language lateralization and dyslexia as an example (Bishop 2013):

1   Endophenotype model: This model assumes that genetic variation in specific risk genes can lead to atypical hemispheric asymmetries that in turn cause a specific symptom, such as language impairment, that is associated with a disorder, such as dyslexia. In this model, atypical lateralization causes the disorder.

2   Neuroplasticity model: This model assumes that genetic variation in specific risk genes can lead to a disorder and that neuroplastic processes associated with this disorder would then cause atypical hemispheric asymmetries. In this model, the disorder causes atypical lateralization.

3   Pleiotropy model: This model assumes that the same genes affect both hemispheric asymmetries and pathogenesis of the disorder but without a causal link between the two.

4   Additive or interactive risks model: This model assumes that certain genes affect the probability of developing a disorder, without affecting hemispheric asymmetries. Atypical hemispheric asymmetries would

then represent an additional risk factor to develop a disorder but again without a causal link between the two.

Which of these four models is best suited to explain the relationship between atypical hemispheric asymmetries and neurodevelopmental disorders? For language lateralization and dyslexia, Bishop (2013) concluded that weak language lateralization likely is a consequence of language disorders like dyslexia, as it is less heritable and less stable than language disorders (see the following). This would support the neuroplasticity model. To assess how these models fit the data, a crucial step is to assess to what extent the genetic determinants of hemispheric asymmetries overlap with those of neurodevelopmental and psychiatric disorders. The first three models all would suggest a substantial overlap between the two, while the last model would not predict such an overlap.

Are there genetic links between hemispheric asymmetries and neurodevelopmental and psychiatric disorders?

In general, the large majority of studies investigating the genetic determinants of hemispheric asymmetries in humans have focused on handedness as phenotype (Güntürkün *et al.* 2020). The largest study to date analysed genetic data from more than 1.7 million individuals obtained from the UK Biobank, 23andMe, and the International Handedness Consortium with handedness phenotypes assessed by questionnaire (Cuellar-Partida *et al.* 2020). Several of the analyses included in this study offered relevant insights in the context of clinical laterality research.

Heritability analysis revealed that additive genetic effects explained 11.9% of the phenotypic variance in handedness, while shared environmental effects accounted for 4.6% and individual environmental effects accounted for 83.6% of the handedness variance. Moreover, a previous large-scale study suggested that genes explain about 24% of the variance in handedness (Medland *et al.* 2009). These findings highlight the importance of taking environmental factors into account when assessing the relation of hemispheric asymmetries and neurodevelopmental and psychiatric disorders.

Interestingly, heritability analyses for language lateralization suggested low heritability for this trait. A recent twin study using functional transcranial Doppler ultrasound to assess the heritability of language lateralization reported that the heritability estimate was zero (Bishop and Bates 2019). Similarly, a dichotic listening family study reported low and non-significant heritability for the right ear advantage in dichotic listening task (Ocklenburg *et al.* 2016a).

In addition to heritability analyses, Cuellar-Partida *et al.* (2020) also performed genome-wide association studies (GWAS) for left-handedness and mixed-handedness. In the left-handedness GWAS, 41 loci reached genome-wide significance. Tissue-enrichment analysis revealed that the central nervous system and especially the brain were relevant for the aetiology of handedness, which is consistent with the idea that handedness is caused by the brain, as it is a form of hemispheric asymmetry. Functionally, the significant loci were involved in the regulation of microtubules and axons, as well as in neurogenesis and morphology regulation of the hippocampus and cortex.

An involvement of microtubule-associated genes, most prominently *MAP2*, in handedness has also been confirmed by two independent GWAS in the UK Biobank dataset (De Kovel and Francks 2019; Wiberg *et al.* 2019). These findings are highly relevant from a clinical laterality perspective for two reasons. First, three single nucleotide polymorphisms that reached significance in the left-handedness GWAS by Cuellar-Partida *et al.* (2020) (rs6224, rs13107325, and rs45527431) had previously been associated with schizophrenia, suggesting a direct overlap between the genetic determinants of handedness and schizophrenia. Importantly, it has been shown that several disorders that have been associated with altered hemispheric asymmetries also show changes in microtubules and/or microtubule-associated proteins (Marchisella *et al.* 2016). Microtubules are polymers that form parts of the cytoskeleton, which has been implicated in setting up cell chirality, a function that is highly important for left-right asymmetric development (Inaki *et al.* 2016). Moreover, it has been suggested that disruption of microtubule function could lead to disruptions in synaptic connectivity which could present a risk factor for the development of neurodevelopmental and psychiatric disorders (Marchisella *et al.* 2016). These include ASD (Chang *et al.* 2018), affective disorders (Gartside *et al.* 2003), and schizophrenia (Prabakaran *et al.* 2004).

In addition to these findings on microtubule-associated genes, a further genetic link between hemispheric asymmetries and neurodevelopmental and psychiatric disorders are genetic pathways involved in the development and function of cilia (Trulioff *et al.* 2017). Cilia are cell organelles that play a part in establishing left/right body asymmetry during development and cilia-associated genes have been related to both hemispheric asymmetries and the pathogenesis of dyslexia (Brandler and Paracchini 2014; Paracchini *et al.* 2016). Besides dyslexia, cilia have been implicated in the pathogenesis of schizophrenia and bipolar disorder (Muñoz-Estrada *et al.* 2018) and ASD (Wang and Brandon 2011).

Taken together, both genetic pathways that link hemispheric asymmetries to neurodevelopmental and psychiatric disorders do so in a diagnosis-unspecific way, as they have been associated with multiple different diagnoses. Moreover, a recent analysis by the Brainstorm consortium revealed many psychiatric disorders show a high degree of genetic correlation, suggesting a deeply interconnected molecular base for these disorders (Anttila *et al.* 2018). This suggests that the link between hemispheric asymmetries and psychopathology might be largely independent of specific diagnoses. Another important insight from the Cuellar-Partida *et al.* (2020) study is that the genetic overlap between hemispheric asymmetries and neurodevelopmental and psychiatric disorders is likely to be moderate but not strong. While three of the loci that reached genome-wide significance for handedness were also associated with schizophrenia, the remaining 38 were not. This makes both the endophenotype and the neuroplasticity model suggested by Bishop (2013) unlikely to fit the data, as both would suggest a more substantial genetic overlap between hemispheric asymmetries and neurodevelopmental and psychiatric disorders. Instead, we argue that it would support a slightly modified version of the pleiotropy model that assumes a partial overlap, similarly to what we have suggested for handedness and language lateralization (Ocklenburg *et al.* 2014). This would suggest a substantial amount of independent ontogenetic influences for the two traits, but also some overlap.

Are there non-genetic links between hemispheric asymmetries and neurodevelopmental and psychiatric disorders?

As lined out previously, the heritability analysis by Cuellar-Partida *et al.* (2020) revealed that only 11.9% of the phenotypic variance in handedness was explained by genetic effects, with the remaining 88.1% percent being explained by environmental factors. This highlights the importance of also taking into account environmental factors when assessing overlaps in the ontogenesis of hemispheric asymmetries and the pathogenesis of neurodevelopmental and psychiatric disorders. Regarding the role of early life factors on the ontogenesis of hemispheric asymmetries, a recent large scale study in the UK Biobank sample found that the probability of being a left-hander was influenced by the year and location of birth, birthweight, being part of a multiple birth, season of birth, breastfeeding and sex (De Kovel *et al.* 2019b). Having a lower birthweight and being part of a multiple birth both increased the probability of atypical hemispheric asymmetry (e.g. being left-handed). Since both having a lower birthweight and being part of a multiple birth have been linked to a higher probability of adverse birth outcomes, preterm birth, and stress in both child and mother (Dunkel Schetter and Tanner 2012; Rondó *et al.* 2003; Torche 2011), it is conceivable that stress hormones could affect hemispheric asymmetries (Ocklenburg *et al.* 2016b). This idea is not without debate, and two large-scale studies preceding the work by De Kovel *et al.* (2019) did not find associations between left-handedness and birth stress or pregnancy risk events (Bailey and McKeever 2004; McManus 1981). Interestingly, a recent review article concluded that there is a strong link between hemispheric asymmetries and maternal stress but only a minor effect of birth complications (Schmitz *et al.* 2017). Moreover, a recent review of the published literature on environmental factors influencing hemispheric asymmetries concluded that of all environmental factors that are associated with hemispheric asymmetries, stress is the only one that has also been substantially linked to psychiatric and neurodevelopmental disorders (Berretz *et al.* 2020).

Stress, hemispheric asymmetries, and psychopathology

The leading pioneer in the investigation of stress and the stress response was Dr Hans Selye (Szabo *et al.* 2012; Selye 1950). He further termed "distress" and "eustress" in the early 1970s to distinguish whether the stress response was initiated by negative, unpleasant stressors, or positive emotions as stress exposure is not harmful per se. Controllable stress, for example, can lead to a positive adaptive modification of brain function and structure. Uncontrollable and psychosocial stress meanwhile can lead to maladaptive changes, especially when experienced in critical periods of brain development (Huether 1996). Nowadays, negative stress exposure is suggested as increasing the risk to develop psychological and physical health problems, including depression, schizophrenia, cancer, and autoimmune disorders (Shields and Slavich 2017).

Generally, the stress response is mainly regulated via the hypothalamic-pituitary-adrenal (HPA)-axis. In brief, secretion of the corticotrophin-releasing hormone (CRH) from hypothalamic paraventricular (PVN) cells results in the release of adrenocorticotropic hormone (ACTH) from the pituitary. ACTH then induces the adrenal cortex to produce glucocorticoids which bind to glucocorticoid and mineralocorticoid receptors. Therewith, glucocorticoids determine the responsiveness of the HPA-axis to stress (Russell and Lightman 2019). Generally, acute stress exposure leading to acute elevation of corticoids can be beneficial for the individual, however, chronic elevation can result in maladaptation and consequently to severe health problems such as psychiatric disorders (Russell and Lightman 2019).

The association of stress and hemispheric asymmetries has been investigated from several different perspectives. These include the role of early life stress (ELS) on the development of hemispheric asymmetries, the effect of stress on functional asymmetries, and the relation of stress and structural hemispheric asymmetries (Ocklenburg *et al.* 2016b; Zach *et al.* 2016). For example, a recent ELS study in rats found that prolonged maternal separation stress leads to more leftward turning behaviour compared to control animals, suggesting a link between ELS and motor asymmetries in rodents (Mundorf *et al.* 2020). For functional asymmetries, it has been suggested that elevated glucocorticoid levels might influence cerebral asymmetries by altering callosal communication between the two hemispheres (Ocklenburg *et al.* 2016b). This often, but not always, results in greater involvement of the right hemisphere, consistent with the idea that the right hemisphere is dominant for the processing of negative emotions which might be elicited by prolonged stress.

Importantly, stress exposure has also been implicated in the pathogenesis of almost all neurodevelopmental and psychiatric disorders, including dyslexia (Kershner 2019), ASD (Beversdorf *et al.* 2018), attention deficit hyperactivity disorder (Fairchild 2012), stuttering (Choi *et al.* 2016), schizophrenia (Howes *et al.* 2017), affective disorders (Ehlert *et al.* 2001), and PTSD (Ehlert *et al.* 2001). Thus, stress is highly relevant for psychopathology but also highly diagnostically unspecific for any single neurodevelopmental or psychiatric disorder. Especially ELS is known to increase the risk for several psychiatric disorders (Carr *et al.* 2013). This is particularly relevant given the high number of adults reporting childhood abuse worldwide (Heim *et al.* 2019). It is proposed that ELS during critical periods of brain development induces long-term neurobiological consequences, especially in regions implicated in regulating emotions and the stress response. This makes stress a core cause of psychiatric disorders (Teicher *et al.* 2003; Lupien *et al.* 2009). Given the HPA-axis as the main stress response, it comes as no surprise that aberrant HPA-axis activity is found in many neurodevelopmental and psychiatric disorders varying in the directionality depending on the disorder. For example, HPA-axis activity is found to be chronically elevated in melancholic depression and schizophrenia and more reactive to stress in social anxiety and ASD. Contrary, HPA-axis activity seems to be low in PTSD and atypical depression (Jacobson 2014).

However, not everybody exposed to adversity in life will develop mental health problems and whether or not someone develops a disorder depends on both genes and environment and most importantly their interaction (Heim *et al.* 2019). The importance of gene-environment interactions in stress exposure and mental health outcome is especially known in depression. For example, it is proposed that a polymorphism in the serotonin transporter gene interacts with adverse life events resulting in HPA-axis hyper-reactivity and, thus, increasing the risk of developing depression (Alexander *et al.* 2009). A promising mechanism to mediate between gene expression and environmental factors such as stress is DNA methylation (Alexander *et al.* 2014). For example, methylation levels of the serotonin transporter gene moderate the association of polymorphisms in this gene and cortisol stress reactivity (Alexander *et al.* 2014). Overall, multiple genes are proposed as mediating between exposure and psychopathology due to DNA methylation changes after exposure (Cecil *et al.* 2020). Interestingly, a recent study also provided tentative evidence for a link between birth stress and methylation in *NEUROD6*, a gene that is asymmetrically expressed in foetal brains (Schmitz *et al.* 2018).

The potential role of stress as an ontogenetic factor influencing both hemispheric asymmetries and potentially all psychiatric and most neurodevelopmental disorders may also explain why there are so many disorders with reduced or reversed hemispheric asymmetries but none with increased hemispheric asymmetries. If the same environmental factor is relevant for atypical hemispheric asymmetries in many or all disorders reviewed in this book, it comes as no surprise that the lateralization patterns are often similar (e.g. higher incidence of non-right-handedness in many disorders).

Transdiagnostic approaches

Taken together, both the genetic and the non-genetic factors that show an overlap between the ontogenesis of hemispheric asymmetries and neurodevelopmental and psychiatric disorders seem to be diagnostically unspecific, as they have been implied in many different disorders. This suggests that transdiagnostic approaches could help conceptualize the relation of hemispheric asymmetries and psychopathology. The clinical classification systems used to diagnose and categorize the disorders described in this book, namely the DSM-5 and ICD-10, imply that mental disorders are distinct, independent, and categorical constructs (Krueger and Eaton 2015). This would mean that a patient either meets the diagnostic threshold for a particular disorder or not (categorical), that there is no overlap with any other mental disorder (distinct), and thus having one disorder does not increase the risk of having any other disorder (independent) (Krueger and Eaton 2015). However, this is not the case on both the behavioural and the genetic level (see the preceding discussion), highlighting the need for new, transdiagnostic approaches using factors such as disorder persistence, age of onset, or an internalizing-externalizing model (Caspi *et al.* 2014; Krueger and Eaton 2015). Besides behavioural categorization, the need for biological parameters to facilitate classification, and thus treatment of disorders, is increasing. However, so far it has been difficult to find disorder-specific alterations as, for example, across multiple disorders, the same genes are implicated (such as the serotonin transporter gene and the glucocorticoid receptor gene) (Cecil *et al.* 2020). These results rather suggest a general dimension of psychopathology, called the p-factor, which directly influences all symptom factors and would also reflect a general risk to develop any or all forms of psychopathology, independent of the disorder (Selzam *et al.* 2018; Caspi *et al.* 2014). This p-factor would also explain why researchers are still struggling to find cause, consequence, biomarkers, and treatments with specificity to individual disorders. Moreover, given the general risk factor of stress exposure and the importance of altered HPA-axis activity across mental disorders, it seems more than likely that all mental disorders share some common biological cause. Whether this cause might be associated with altered atypical asymmetries is still to be investigated.

Within the context of transdiagnostic approaches, one research framework that has been suggested to be relevant for the relation of hemispheric asymmetries and psychopathology is the Research Domain Criteria (RDoC) framework (Insel *et al.* 2010). RDoC reconceptualizes mental health and illness by focusing on distinct symptom domains, such as negative valence, positive valence, social and arousal systems, instead of distinct disorder diagnoses. Applying such a research framework in clinical laterality research may be helpful, as several studies reviewed in the previous chapters suggested that symptom severity and not diagnosis per se is the critical factor in whether or not an individual shows atypical asymmetries in, for example, schizophrenia (Ocklenburg *et al.* 2013) or dyslexia (Helland *et al.* 2008). A study using an RDoC perspective for investigating the relation of frontal electroencephalographic asymmetries to affective and anxiety-related symptoms (Nusslock *et al.* 2015) found that frontal electroencephalogram (EEG) asymmetries were associated with specific symptom clusters, such as anhedonia, excessive approach motivation, and anxious apprehension. This highlights that moving beyond distinct diagnoses and using a symptom-based approach should be considered when designing future clinical laterality studies, as has been recently suggested for laterality research in schizophrenia (Ocklenburg *et al.* 2015).

Conclusion

In conclusion, it is unlikely that atypical hemispheric asymmetries are the cause of neurodevelopmental and psychiatric disorders (Bishop 2013). Conversely, it is also unlikely that altered hemispheric asymmetries are a causal effect of neurodevelopment and psychiatric disorders. Both models would suggest a stronger overlap between the ontogenetic influence factors for these two traits. Instead, the empirical evidence presented in this chapter makes it conceivable that several ontogenetic pathways influence both hemispheric asymmetries and neurodevelopmental and psychiatric disorders but that there are also a substantial number of independent influence factors. On the genetic side, these pathways include the development and function of cilia as well as the development and function of microtubules. On the environmental side, stress seems to affect both hemispheric asymmetries and pathogenesis of almost all neurodevelopmental and psychiatric disorders. Importantly, both stress and the two genetic pathways seem to be diagnostically unspecific, as they have been implied in many different disorders. This could explain why so many different disorders show a change of hemispheric asymmetries in the same direction and highlight the importance of transdiagnostic symptom-based approaches for future clinical laterality studies.

The importance of open science in clinical laterality research

The replication crisis

The term replication crisis refers to the fact that both basic and clinical psychological research have low replication rates, for example, published findings often do not replicate when the same experiment is performed in a different lab (Tackett et al. 2019). In 2015, the Open Science Collaboration conducted replications of 100 published psychological studies using design with high statistical power. While 97% of the original studies reported statistically significant effects, only 36% of the replication studies observed statistically significant results (Open Science Collaboration 2015). Moreover, effect sizes showed a substantial decline with replication effects having only half the magnitude of original effects. While the causes for the replication crisis are difficult to disentangle, several factors that likely contribute to replication issues have been identified. These include the fact that psychological studies are often statistically underpowered due to small sample sizes and the fact that there are often a high number of tested relationships but only statistically significant ones are reported. Moreover, researchers have a personal interest in obtaining significant effects to get publications that are relevant for advancing their careers (Ioannidis 2005). Here, specifically, a culture that expects researchers to acquire external funding to get tenure has been criticized for providing incentive to engage in questionable research practices to obtain significant results (Lilienfeld 2017).

Clinical laterality research and the replication crisis

Given the fact that less than 50% of significant results replicate, it comes as no surprise that a 2020 article discussing the research trends that are likely to shape laterality research in the next decade identified finding laterality-specific solutions to the replication crisis as one of these trends (Ocklenburg *et al.* 2020). As in any other field of research, there are examples in clinical laterality research in which overblown claims based on underpowered samples did not replicate in subsequent studies. The most widely discussed example in this regard is in all likelihood a 1988 study published in the prestigious scientific journal, *Nature* (Halpern and Coren 1988). The authors claimed that right-handers live significantly longer than left-handers based on analysing the mean age of death of 1472 right-handed and 236 left-handed baseball players from a book titled *The Baseball Encyclopedia*. In 1991, the authors of the baseball study followed up with a study in *The New England Journal of Medicine* analysing the death certificates of 987 people from California, this time claiming that left-handers die nine years earlier than right-handers (Halpern and Coren 1991). However, these findings were widely discussed and failed to replicate (Harris 1993; McManus 2019). Most recently, McManus analysed the death rates of left- and right-handers in the UK Biobank (McManus 2019). In this databank, 500,000 individuals were tested, a number that was substantially larger than the datasets analysed in both studies by Halpern and Coren. McManus (2019) reported that the relative mortality of left-handers compared to right-handers in this cohort was almost exactly 1.0, indicating no differences in longevity between left- and right-handers.

While such obvious cases are rare, replication issues are likely to affect clinical laterality research on a much wider level. One example comes from the data on structural asymmetries in affective disorders discussed in Chapter 3 of this book. In this field, an early neuroimaging study investigated structural hemispheric asymmetries in grey matter volume in a sample of 52 depressed patients and 30 controls and reported reduced frontal lobe asymmetries in the depressed patients (Kumar *et al.* 2000). Subsequently, a study in a substantially larger sample of 70 patients with major depressive disorder (MDD) and 349 healthy controls reported that depressed patients showed a significantly reduced volumetric asymmetry in the dorsolateral prefrontal cortex that was associated with depressive symptoms (Liu *et al.* 2016). The largest study so far on altered structural hemispheric asymmetries in grey matter in depression was conducted by the ENIGMA consortium and had an overall sample size of 2256 patients with MDD and 3503 control subjects (De Kovel *et al.* 2019a). In contrast to the earlier studies, no difference in volumetric asymmetries of 34 cortical and 8 subcortical brain regions was observed. This non-replication of the earlier significant findings in the largest investigated dataset so far highlights the importance of large-scale datasets in clinical laterality research. It is difficult to estimate to what extent clinical laterality research, in general, is affected by replication issues.

A non-clinical replication study investigating the reproducibility of nine different published results that were obtained with the divided visual field paradigm (Brederoo *et al.* 2019) found precise and reliable evidence supporting visual field asymmetries in five categories (faces, emotions, global/local information, word, and spatial attention). Less convincing evidence was found for visual field asymmetries in processing of high and low spatial frequencies, and no evidence for visual field asymmetries was found for oddball perception and categorical and coordinate spatial judgments. This suggests that, in general, the reproducibility in laterality research might be somewhat higher than the 37% reported by the Open Science Collaboration (2015).

Solutions to the replication crisis in clinical laterality research

If clinical laterality research is indeed affected by the replication crisis, what can be done to identify effects that replicate reliably and foster reproducible and transparent research for future projects? Altogether, three main solutions for these issues have been brought forward.

First, meta-analytic integration of published datasets is a key technique to solve one of the key issues of the replication crisis: low statistical power due to low cohort sizes. Patient cohorts are often difficult to recruit resulting in low cohort sizes. This is a major problem, especially since the dependent variables in clinical laterality research often have heavily skewed distributions. For example, for handedness, it has been found that 10.6% of people are left-handed and 89.4% are right-handed (Papadatou-Pastou *et al.* 2020). If handedness is the dependent variable in a clinical laterality study, substantial cohort sizes are paramount to detect effects. Therefore, several meta-analyses have been conducted on handedness in clinical samples in, for example, ASD (Markou *et al.* 2017) or schizophrenia (Hirnstein and Hugdahl 2014), as discussed in the previous chapters. In contrast, meta-analytic integration of differences between clinical groups and controls in other laterality measures, such as dichotic listening performance or frontal EEG alpha asymmetries, are mostly still lacking and should be performed in the future. In addition to classical meta-analyses that typically compare effect sizes between two groups such as patients and controls, activation likelihood estimation (ALE) meta-analysis that determine brain activation convergence between different neuroimaging studies (Eickhoff *et al.* 2012) have seen increasing use in clinical laterality research over the last decades as described in the previous chapters. ALE meta-analysis is a powerful tool that allows determination of lateralization differences between clinical groups and controls on a regional level and of which brain regions show replicable differences in laterality between two groups. Therefore, ALE should be used to investigate lateralization of brain activation in clinical groups in which it has not been used so far.

Both ALE meta-analyses and classic meta-analyses, however, have two major issues. On the one hand, they are affected by publication bias (Egger *et al.* 2001), the tendency that scientific results that are statistically significant have a higher chance of getting published. Thus, if significant results are more likely to get published and non-significant results are more likely to end up non-published, a meta-analysis might overestimate true effect sizes. Moreover, the scientific quality of the integrated studies affects the scientific quality of the meta-analysis. If only low-quality studies are integrated into a meta-analysis, the results of this meta-analysis might not be very replicable. Therefore, a meta-analysis of existing data should be supplemented by new data collection in multi-lab large-scale studies and analysis of databanks that contain laterality data, such as the UK Biobank. For clinical laterality research, such studies have mostly been conducted by the ENIGMA consortium (Kong *et al.* 2020), for example in ASD (Postema *et al.* 2019) and depression (De Kovel *et al.* 2019a). These two examples also beautifully exemplify the importance of such large-scale studies. For both ASD and depression, previous studies have reported alterations of grey-matter volume asymmetries between the clinical group and controls. While the ENIGMA ASD study showed evidence for differences in structural brain asymmetries in several regions, no differences were observed in the ENIGMA depression study. Therefore, results reported in small sample empirical studies do not have a high predictive value for what will be observed in large-scale studies. Taken together, conducting more such large-scale multi-lab studies on laterality in clinical groups is highly important.

Obviously, not all studies can test effects in cohorts of several thousand participants. When clinical laterality studies can only be conducted in smaller cohorts, following the principles of open science in laterality research as outlined in the recently published roadmap for the journal *Laterality* (Grimshaw *et al.* 2020), is essential. This includes, for example, the publication of registered reports in which stage one manuscripts including the introduction, method, and planned analyses get accepted independent of whether or not the authors report significant effects or not. Afterward, the authors conduct the research and then submit a stage-two manuscript which gets reviewed without taking the significance of results into account. This way of publishing scientific data is essential in reducing publication bias. Moreover, data and analysis code should be openly available on platforms, such as the Open Science Framework or others, to enhance transparency and reproducibility of analyses.

Conclusion

It is difficult to pinpoint to which extent clinical laterality research has been impacted by the replication crisis. Based on the comparison of large-scale and small-scale studies on structural asymmetries, we can assume that there are several published effects in clinical laterality that are unlikely to replicate. The next decade will hopefully bring more large-scale studies and meta-analyses along with the widespread implementation of the principles of open science in smaller studies. We are confident that such measures will lead to an increase in transparency and reproducibility in this fascinating area of neuroscience.

References

Alexander, N., *et al.*, 2009. Gene-environment interactions predict cortisol responses after acute stress: implications for the etiology of depression. *Psychoneuroendocrinology*, 34 (9), 1294–1303.

Alexander, N., *et al.*, 2014. DNA methylation profiles within the serotonin transporter gene moderate the association of 5-HTTLPR and cortisol stress reactivity. *Translational Psychiatry*, 4, e443.

Anttila, V., *et al.*, 2018. Analysis of shared heritability in common disorders of the brain. *Science (New York, N.Y.)*, 360 (6395).

Bailey, L.M., and McKeever, W.F., 2004. A large-scale study of handedness and pregnancy/birth risk events: implications for genetic theories of handedness. *Laterality*, 9 (2), 175–188.

Banmen, J., 1983. Cerebral laterality and its implications for psychotherapy. *International Journal for the Advancement of Counselling*, 6 (2), 99–113.

Berretz, G., *et al.*, 2020. Atypical lateralization in neurodevelopmental and psychiatric disorders: what is the role of stress? *Cortex*, 125, 215–232.

Beversdorf, D.Q., Stevens, H.E., and Jones, K.L., 2018. Prenatal stress, maternal immune dysregulation, and their association with autism spectrum disorders. *Current Psychiatry Reports*, 20 (9), 76.

Bishop, D.V.M., 2013. Cerebral asymmetry and language development: cause, correlate, or consequence? *Science (New York, N.Y.)*, 340 (6138), 1230531.

Bishop, D.V.M., and Bates, T.C., 2019. Heritability of language laterality assessed by functional transcranial Doppler ultrasound: a twin study. *Wellcome Open Research*, 4, 161.

Brandler, W.M., and Paracchini, S., 2014. The genetic relationship between handedness and neurodevelopmental disorders. *Trends in Molecular Medicine*, 20 (2), 83–90.

Brederoo, S.G., *et al.*, 2019. Reproducibility of visual-field asymmetries: nine replication studies investigating lateralization of visual information processing. *Cortex*, 111, 100–126.

Bruder, G., 1996. Dichotic listening before and after fluoxetine treatment for major depression: relations of laterality to therapeutic response. *Neuropsychopharmacology: Official Publication of the American College of Neuropsychopharmacology*, 15 (2), 171–179.

Bruder, G.E., *et al.*, 2004. Dichotic listening tests of functional brain asymmetry predict response to fluoxetine in depressed women and men. *Neuropsychopharmacology: Official Publication of the American College of Neuropsychopharmacology*, 29 (9), 1752–1761.

Carr, C.P., *et al.*, 2013. The role of early life stress in adult psychiatric disorders: a systematic review according to childhood trauma subtypes. *The Journal of Nervous and Mental Disease*, 201 (12), 1007–1020.

Caspi, A., *et al.*, 2014. The p factor: one general psychopathology factor in the structure of psychiatric disorders? *Clinical Psychological Science: A Journal of the Association for Psychological Science*, 2 (2), 119–137.

Cecil, C.A., Zhang, Y., and Nolte, T., 2020. Childhood maltreatment and DNA methylation: a systematic review. *Neuroscience & Biobehavioral Reviews*, 112, 392–409.

Chang, Q., *et al.*, 2018. Role of microtubule-associated protein in autism spectrum disorder. *Neuroscience Bulletin*, 34 (6), 1119–1126.

Choi, D., *et al.*, 2016. Emotional diathesis, emotional stress, and childhood stuttering. *Journal of Speech, Language, and Hearing Research: JSLHR*, 59 (4), 616–630.

Cuellar-Partida, G., *et al.*, 2020. Genome-wide association study identifies 48 common genetic variants associated with handedness. *Nature Human Behaviour*, 5, 59–70.

De Kovel, Carolien G.F., *et al.*, 2019a. No alterations of brain structural asymmetry in major depressive disorder: an ENIGMA consortium analysis. *The American Journal of Psychiatry*, 176 (12), 1039–1049.

De Kovel, Carolien G.F., Carrión-Castillo, A., and Francks, C., 2019b. A large-scale population study of early life factors influencing left-handedness. *Scientific Reports*, 9 (1), 584.

De Kovel, Carolien G.F., and Francks, C., 2019. The molecular genetics of hand preference revisited. *Scientific Reports*, 9 (1), 5986.

Dunkel Schetter, C., and Tanner, L., 2012. Anxiety, depression and stress in pregnancy: implications for mothers, children, research, and practice. *Current Opinion in Psychiatry*, 25 (2), 141–148.

Egger, M., Smith, G.D., and Sterne, J.A., 2001. Uses and abuses of meta-analysis. *Clinical Medicine (London, England)*, 1 (6), 478–484.

Ehlert, U., Gaab, J., and Heinrichs, M., 2001. Psychoneuroendocrinological contributions to the etiology of depression, posttraumatic stress disorder, and stress-related bodily disorders: the role of the hypothalamus-pituitary-adrenal axis. *Biological Psychology*, 57 (1–3), 141–152.

Eickhoff, S.B., *et al.*, 2012. Activation likelihood estimation meta-analysis revisited. *NeuroImage*, 59 (3), 2349–2361.

Fairchild, G., 2012. Hypothalamic-pituitary-adrenocortical axis function in atten-tion-deficit hyperactivity disorder. *Current Topics in Behavioral Neurosciences*, 9, 93–111.

Forbes, D., *et al.*, 2006. Is mixed-handedness a marker of treatment response in posttraumatic stress disorder?: a pilot study. *Journal of Traumatic Stress*, 19 (6), 961–966.

Gartside, S.E., *et al.*, 2003. Flattening the glucocorticoid rhythm causes changes in hippocampal expression of messenger RNAs coding structural and functional proteins: implications for aging and depression. *Neuropsychopharmacology: Official Publication of the American College of Neuropsychopharmacology*, 28 (5), 821–829.

Grimshaw, G., Hausmann, M., and Rogers, L., 2020. A new roadmap for laterality: asymmetries of brain, behaviour, and cognition. *Laterality*, 25 (1), 1–4.

Güntürkün, O., Ströckens, F., and Ocklenburg, S., 2020. Brain lateralization: a com-parative perspective. *Physiological Reviews*, 100 (3), 1019–1063.

Halpern, D.F., and Coren, S., 1988. Do right-handers live longer? *Nature*, 333 (6170), 213.

Halpern, D.F., and Coren, S., 1991. Handedness and life span. *The New England Journal of Medicine*, 324 (14), 998.

Harris, L.J., 1993. Do left-handers die sooner than right-handers? Commentary on Coren and Halpern's (1991) "Left-handedness: a marker for decreased survival fitness". *Psychological Bulletin*, 114 (2), 203–234; discussion 235–247.

Heim, C.M., Entringer, S., and Buss, C., 2019. Translating basic research knowl-edge on the biological embedding of early-life stress into novel approaches for the developmental programming of lifelong health. *Psychoneuroendocrinology*, 105, 123–137.

Helland, T., *et al.*, 2008. Dichotic listening and school performance in dyslexia. *Dyslexia (Chichester, England)*, 14 (1), 42–53.

Hirnstein, M., and Hugdahl, K., 2014. Excess of non-right-handedness in schizo-phrenia: meta-analysis of gender effects and potential biases in handedness assessment. *The British Journal of Psychiatry: The Journal of Mental Science*, 205 (4), 260–267.

Howes, O.D., *et al.*, 2017. The role of genes, stress, and dopamine in the develop-ment of schizophrenia. *Biological Psychiatry*, 81 (1), 9–20.

Huether, G., 1996. The central adaptation syndrome: psychosocial stress as a trig-ger for adaptive modifications of brain structure and brain function. *Progress in Neurobiology*, 48 (6), 569–612.

Inaki, M., Liu, J., and Matsuno, K., 2016. Cell chirality: its origin and roles in left-right asymmetric development. *Philosophical Transactions of the Royal Society of London. Series B, Biological Sciences*, 371 (1710).

Insel, T., *et al.*, 2010. Research domain criteria (RDoC): toward a new classification framework for research on mental disorders. *The American Journal of Psychiatry*, 167 (7), 748–751.

Ioannidis, J.P.A., 2005. Why most published research findings are false. *PLoS Medi-cine*, 2 (8), e124.

Jacobson, L., 2014. Hypothalamic-pituitary-adrenocortical axis: neuropsychiatric aspects. *Comprehensive Physiology*, 4 (2), 715–738.

Kershner, J.R., 2019. Neurobiological systems in dyslexia. *Trends in Neuroscience and Education*, 14, 11–24.

Kishon, R., *et al.*, 2015. Lateralization for speech predicts therapeutic response to cognitive behavioral therapy for depression. *Psychiatry Research*, 228 (3), 606–611.

Kong, X.-Z., *et al.*, 2020. Mapping brain asymmetry in health and disease through the ENIGMA consortium. *Human Brain Mapping*, Online ahead of print.

Krueger, R.F., and Eaton, N.R., 2015. Transdiagnostic factors of mental disorders. *World Psychiatry: Official Journal of the World Psychiatric Association (WPA)*, 14 (1), 27–29.

Kumar, A., *et al.*, 2000. Volumetric asymmetries in late-onset mood disorders: an attenuation of frontal asymmetry with depression severity. *Psychiatry Research: Neuroimaging*, 100 (1), 41–47.

Lilienfeld, S.O., 2017. Psychology's replication crisis and the grant culture: righting the ship. *Perspectives on Psychological Science: A Journal of the Association for Psychological Science*, 12 (4), 660–664.

Liu, W., *et al.*, 2016. Structural asymmetry of dorsolateral prefrontal cortex correlates with depressive symptoms: evidence from healthy individuals and patients with major depressive disorder. *Neuroscience Bulletin*, 32 (3), 217–226.

Lupien, S.J., *et al.*, 2009. Effects of stress throughout the lifespan on the brain, behaviour and cognition. *Nature Reviews. Neuroscience*, 10 (6), 434–445.

Marchisella, F., Coffey, E.T., and Hollos, P., 2016. Microtubule and microtubule associated protein anomalies in psychiatric disease. *Cytoskeleton (Hoboken, N.J.)*, 73 (10), 596–611.

Markou, P., Ahtam, B., and Papadatou-Pastou, M., 2017. Elevated levels of atypical handedness in autism: meta-analyses. *Neuropsychology Review*, 27 (3), 258–283.

McManus, I.C., 1981. Handedness and birth stress. *Psychological Medicine*, 11 (3), 485–496.

McManus, I.C., 2019. Half a century of handedness research: myths, truths; fictions, facts; backwards, but mostly forwards. *Brain and Neuroscience Advances*, 3, 2398212818820513.

Medland, S.E., *et al.*, 2009. Genetic influences on handedness: data from 25,732 Australian and Dutch twin families. *Neuropsychologia*, 47 (2), 330–337.

Mundorf, A., *et al.*, 2020. Asymmetry of turning behavior in rats is modulated by early life stress. *Behavioural Brain Research*, 393, 112807.

Muñoz-Estrada, J., *et al.*, 2018. Primary cilia formation is diminished in schizophrenia and bipolar disorder: a possible marker for these psychiatric diseases. *Schizophrenia Research*, 195, 412–420.

Nusslock, R., Walden, K., and Harmon-Jones, E., 2015. Asymmetrical frontal cortical activity associated with differential risk for mood and anxiety disorder symptoms: an RDoC perspective. *International Journal of Psychophysiology: Official Journal of the International Organization of Psychophysiology*, 98 (2 Pt 2), 249–261.

Ocklenburg, S., *et al.*, 2013. Auditory hallucinations and reduced language laterali-zation in schizophrenia: a meta-analysis of dichotic listening studies. *Journal of the International Neuropsychological Society: JINS*, 19 (4), 410–418.

Ocklenburg, S., *et al.*, 2014. The ontogenesis of language lateralization and its rela-tion to handedness. *Neuroscience and Biobehavioral Reviews*, 43, 191–198.

Ocklenburg, S., *et al.*, 2015. Laterality and mental disorders in the postgenomic age—a closer look at schizophrenia and language lateralization. *Neuroscience and Biobehavioral Reviews*, 59, 100–110.

Ocklenburg, S., *et al.*, 2016a. Investigating heritability of laterality and cognitive control in speech perception. *Brain and Cognition*, 109, 34–39.

Ocklenburg, S., *et al.*, 2016b. Stress and laterality—the comparative perspective. *Physiology & Behavior*, 164 (Pt A), 321–329.

Ocklenburg, S., *et al.*, 2020. Laterality 2020: entering the next decade. *Laterality*, 1–33.

Oertel-Knöchel, V., *et al.*, 2012. Abnormal functional and structural asymmetry as biomarker for schizophrenia. *Current Topics in Medicinal Chemistry*, 12 (21), 2434–2451.

Open Science Collaboration, 2015. Estimating the reproducibility of psychological science. *Science (New York, N.Y.)*, 349 (6251), aac4716.

Papadatou-Pastou, M., *et al.*, 2020. Human handedness: a meta-analysis. *Psycho-logical Bulletin*, 146 (6), 481–524.

Paracchini, S., Diaz, R., and Stein, J., 2016. Advances in dyslexia genetics-new insights into the role of brain asymmetries. *Advances in Genetics*, 96, 53–97.

Postema, M.C., *et al.*, 2019. Altered structural brain asymmetry in autism spectrum disorder in a study of 54 datasets. *Nature Communications*, 10 (1), 4958.

Prabakaran, S., *et al.*, 2004. Mitochondrial dysfunction in schizophrenia: evidence for compromised brain metabolism and oxidative stress. *Molecular Psychiatry*, 9 (7), 684–697, 643.

Rondó, P.H.C., *et al.*, 2003. Maternal psychological stress and distress as predictors of low birth weight, prematurity and intrauterine growth retardation. *European Journal of Clinical Nutrition*, 57 (2), 266–272.

Russell, G., and Lightman, S., 2019. The human stress response. *Nature Reviews. Endocrinology*, 15 (9), 525–534.

Satz, P., 1972. Pathological left-handedness: an explanaory model. *Cortex*, 8 (2), 121–135.

Schmitz, J., *et al.*, 2017. Beyond the genome-towards an epigenetic understanding of handedness ontogenesis. *Progress in Neurobiology*, 159, 69–89.

Schmitz, J., *et al.*, 2018. DNA methylation in candidate genes for handedness pre-dicts handedness direction. *Laterality*, 23 (4), 441–461.

Schore, A.N., 2019. *Right brain psychotherapy*. New York: W. W. Norton & Company.

Selye, H., 1950. *The physiology and pathology of exposure to stress*. Oxford, Eng-land: Acta, Inc.

Selzam, S., *et al.*, 2018. A polygenic p factor for major psychiatric disorders. *Trans-lational Psychiatry*, 8 (1), 205.

Shields, G.S., and Slavich, G.M., 2017. Lifetime stress exposure and health: a review of contemporary assessment methods and biological mechanisms. *Social and Personality Psychology Compass*, 11 (8).

Szabo, S., Tache, Y., and Somogyi, A., 2012. The legacy of Hans Selye and the origins of stress research: a retrospective 75 years after his landmark brief "letter" to the editor# of nature. *Stress (Amsterdam, Netherlands)*, 15 (5), 472–478.

Tackett, J.L., *et al.*, 2019. Psychology's replication crisis and clinical psychological science. *Annual Review of Clinical Psychology*, 15, 579–604.

Teicher, M.H., *et al.*, 2003. The neurobiological consequences of early stress and childhood maltreatment. *Neuroscience and Biobehavioral Reviews*, 27 (1–2), 33–44.

Torche, F., 2011. The effect of maternal stress on birth outcomes: exploiting a natural experiment. *Demography*, 48 (4), 1473–1491.

Trulioff, A., Ermakov, A., and Malashichev, Y., 2017. Primary cilia as a possible link between left-right asymmetry and neurodevelopmental diseases. *Genes*, 8 (2).

Wang, Q., and Brandon, N.J., 2011. Regulation of the cytoskeleton by disrupted-in-schizophrenia 1 (DISC1). *Molecular and Cellular Neurosciences*, 48 (4), 359–364.

Weinland, C., *et al.*, 2019. Crossed eye/hand laterality and left-eyedness predict a positive 24-month outcome in alcohol-dependent patients. *Alcoholism, Clinical and Experimental Research*, 43 (6), 1308–1317.

Wiberg, A., *et al.*, 2019. Handedness, language areas and neuropsychiatric diseases: insights from brain imaging and genetics. *Brain: A Journal of Neurology*, 142 (10), 2938–2947.

Zach, P., *et al.*, 2016. Effect of stress on structural brain asymmetry. *Neuro Endocrinology Letters*, 37 (4), 253–264.

Index